The Cleveland Clinic Guide to

ARTHRITIS

The Cleveland Clinic Guide to
ARTHRITIS

John D. Clough, MD

KAPLAN)

PUBLISHING

New York

© 2009 Kaplan Publishing

Artwork is reprinted with the permission of The Cleveland Clinic Center for Medical Art & Photograph © 2009.

Published by Kaplan Publishing, a division of Kaplan, Inc.
1 Liberty Plaza, 24th Floor
New York, NY 10006

Printed in the United States of America

Library of Congress Cataloging-in-Publication Data

Clough, John D.
The Cleveland Clinic guide to arthritis / John D. Clough.
    p. cm.
Includes index.
ISBN 978-1-4277-9956-2

1. Arthritis--Popular works. I. Cleveland Clinic Foundation. II. Title.
RC933.C594 2009
616.7'22--dc22

2008048321

10 9 8 7 6 5 4 3 2 1

ISBN-13: 978-1-4277-9956-2

Kaplan Publishing books are available at special quantity discounts to use for sales promotions, employee premiums, or educational purposes. Please email our Special Sales Department to order or for more information at *kaplanpublishing@kaplan.com,* or write to Kaplan Publishing, 1 Liberty Plaza, 24th Floor, New York, NY 10006.

Contents

Introduction

It has been said that there are more than 100 types of arthritis. While that may be something of an exaggeration, it is nonetheless clear that many types exist. Figuring out what type of arthritis a person has carries important implications, both for assessing the risk of disability and for successfully treating that person.

Arthritis is a common and thoroughly miserable group of conditions. The most recent statistics suggest that about 46.4 million Americans (about 21 percent of the population) of all ages suffer from some kind of arthritis. I've written this book in order to provide some encouragement in seeking treatment, information on some of the most common types of arthritis, and advice on how to cope if you are suffering from one of these ailments. If you have, think you have, or know someone who has arthritis, I hope that you will find some comfort and useful information in these pages.

Many people, upon receiving a diagnosis of arthritis, are surprised to learn how common it is, how many forms of it exist, and that it so frequently begins in young people. There are several reasons for this. Mild or early arthritis, though it is noticeable enough to the person who has it, often is not apparent to the casual observer. Although many types of arthritis are non-destructive, the more damaging forms may take years to cause the more obvious deformities and disabilities we normally associate with arthritis. And the most common type of arthritis—osteoarthritis—really is more typically a disease of the elderly than are many of the other forms.

Notwithstanding the wide diversity of arthritic conditions, it is noteworthy that more than 95 percent of arthritis sufferers have one of the ten or so most common types of arthritis, which we review in this book. We'll also take a look at a couple of very common nonarthritic conditions that are often mistaken for arthritis: fibromyalgia and polymyalgia rheumatica.

In my 43 years of working as a rheumatologist with arthritis patients, I've encountered stories both typical and unusual. Here in this book, you will find each of the conditions explored via case studies of people just like you—people who are in early or advanced stages of arthritis or an arthritis-like condition and who came to the Cleveland Clinic for help.

Founded in 1921, the Cleveland Clinic has evolved into a comprehensive provider of specialty medical and surgical care. Dr. Arthur Scherbel, who founded the institution's rheumatology program in 1953, was interested in treating rheumatoid arthritis aggressively He was one of the first physicians in the world to use drugs normally used to treat cancer, including methotrexate, to treat this disease, beginning in the early 1960s. I joined the department in 1971 with a background in immunology acquired in the immunopathology section of the National Cancer Institute's metabolism branch as a protégé of Dr. Warren Strober. I headed the Cleveland Clinic's rheumatology department from 1979 to 1991, when Dr. Gary Hoffman, a vasculitis expert from the National Institutes of Health, succeeded me. *U.S. News & World Report* ranked the Cleveland Clinic's rheumatology program second in the nation in its 2008 rankings.

The case descriptions in this book are derived from my experiences taking care of arthritis patients at the Cleveland Clinic. Although the patients' names are fictitious, their stories are not, and their responses to treatment are likewise real. As you read these stories, remember that every patient is different, and what works for one does not work for all. Nowhere in medicine is the phrase "One man's meat is another man's poison" more relevant than in arthritis. This book may help to point you in the right direction, but it is no substitute for an experienced, knowledge-able physician. The role of the physician is to help you sift through all of the variation and complexity, come to the right conclusions about diagnosis and treatment, and ultimately get as good an outcome as possible

John D. Clough, M.D.
Cleveland Clinic
Emeritus Staff Rheumatologist

Chapter 1

What's All This about Arthritis?

Do your joints hurt? Are they stiff? Are they swollen? Are they deformed?

Are your muscles weak or sore?

Do you stiffen up after sitting for more than a few minutes?

Are you tired all the time? Do you feel old and decrepit beyond your years?

Do you find yourself eating aspirin or ibuprofen on a regular basis?

If the answer to any or all of these questions is yes, it's possible that you are suffering from arthritis or an arthritis-related condition.

What Is Arthritis?

Arthritis is a word with a very specific meaning, unlike the ambiguous term *rheumatism,* which to most people means aches and pains in the musculoskeletal system. Arthritis means inflammation in one or more joints. Aching and stiffness do not necessarily indicate that you have arthritis, and, by the same token, arthritis isn't just pain in the joints. There must be some additional evidence of inflammation, such as swelling, redness, tenderness, stiffness, or unusual warmth, and it must actually be in the joints, not just in muscles or other surrounding tissues.

Joint pain in itself doesn't equate to arthritis; nevertheless, arthritis is usually painful. The severity may range from moderate and merely annoying to severe and excruciating. Pain is seldom completely absent from an inflamed joint if the sensory nerves serving the joint are normal. In most cases of arthritis, pain is the dominant symptom, though not the only one, especially early on. Later, particularly if untreated, patients may suffer from increasing levels of disability.

• • • *Fast Fact* • • •

The medical term for joint pain is arthralgia. Although pain in the joints typically accompanies arthritis, joint paint alone is not arthritis.

• • •

Although many arthritis sufferers have aching muscles (myalgia) and sore tendons (tendinitis) or bursas, which are fluid sacs that cushion tendons and muscles that would otherwise rub on joints during movements (bursitis), these maladies are not arthritis. They represent different forms of rheumatism that may or may not occur along with arthritis. What makes arthritis more significant than these other forms—painful though they may be—is the potential for it to lead in some cases to joint destruction and permanent disability. Once arthritis has damaged a joint, clearing up the inflammation does not return the joint to a normal state. It's critical to recognize arthritis early and treat it aggressively before damage occurs.

Arthritis should not be thought of as a disease but rather as a symptom that is common to many diseases. When arthritis is the most prominent symptom of the disease it happens to be a part of, the disease is often known as a form of arthritis; for example, rheumatoid arthritis is a systemic disease (rheumatoid disease) that prominently involves the joints, along with other tissues. But many diseases that feature arthritis as a component are not called arthritis. Systemic lupus erythematosus is a prime example. The majority of people with lupus have arthritis as one symptom, but the disease is not primarily thought of as a form of arthritis, probably because its involvement of organs other than the joints—for example, the kidneys and the central nervous system—can be much more serious than the joint involvement in lupus.

Are There Many Kinds of Arthritis?

The most common forms of arthritis are rheumatoid arthritis and osteoarthritis. But there are many other kinds, most of which are not nearly as familiar. This book will examine in some detail several different forms of arthritis and review their distinguishing features.

The National Arthritis Data Workgroup estimates that arthritis causes disability for 19 million people. It leads to 744,000

Arthritis is a common problem. The table below shows that the various forms of arthritis affect more than 46 million people in the United States.

Diagnosis	Americans Afflicted
Osteoarthritis	26.9 million
Gout	6.1 million
Rheumatoid arthritis	1.3 million
Seronegative spondyloarthropathies (including ankylosing spondylitis and psoriatic arthritis)	639,000 to 2.42 million
Juvenile forms of arthritis	188,000 to 400,000
Systemic lupus erythematosus	161,000 to 322,000

hospitalizations and 9,367 deaths annually. It costs the U.S. economy more than $128 billion each year. It is clearly an important problem, both medically and economically. But those numbers only hint at the human misery arthritis causes.

In some cases, arthritis is not even the most threatening manifestation of the disease that causes it, although it often demands the greatest attention because of the pain that accompanies it. Arthritis may be the most prominent early manifestation of such varied diseases as lung cancer, systemic lupus erythematosus, hepatitis, rheumatic fever, tuberculosis, AIDS, and a host of other nasty afflictions. Making the right diagnosis and treating the underlying disease offer the best chance of successfully managing these types of arthritis. Clues suggesting the correct diagnosis can be found in such simple things as:

- Which joints (and how many) are affected

- The length of time and the frequency of joint involvement (intermittent versus constant, acute versus gradual onset, and other similar parameters)

- The amount of pain, tenderness, stiffness, and swelling, as well as relevant abnormalities in areas of the body other than the joints—for instance, skin rashes, hair loss, mouth sores, fever, and nodules under the skin

Although a skilled physician can usually tell with considerable confidence what is going on from these clues, additional information from the laboratory and X-ray departments may help nail down the diagnosis.

What Happens If I Have Arthritis?

Outcomes vary. The diverse forms of arthritis are, in most cases, chronic conditions for which there are no known cures. Even joint infections successfully treated and cured with antibiotics often leave enough residual damage in the affected joints to be chronically problematic thereafter. So a "satisfactory" outcome is a relative thing, depending on the type of arthritis, the stage of the disease when treatment is begun, your willingness and ability to tolerate and persevere in treatment, your activity levels, and other health factors.

It's important for you and your doctor to establish appropriate expectations and time frames when you undergo treatment. While an arthritis diagnosis is no reason to panic, you must be realistic; in most cases, you won't be able to simply take a pill or have surgery and never suffer or worry about pain again. Nevertheless, many people with arthritis live happy and productive lives through a combination of understanding and accommodating to the limitations imposed by the disease along with the appropriate use of medical, surgical, and other treatments.

Should I See a Specialist?

Ideally, the overall treatment programs for people with arthritis should be planned, supervised, and in some cases monitored by specially trained physicians called rheumatologists. If you think you have arthritis, make an appointment with your internist or family physician as soon as possible so that you can ask for a referral. Your primary-care physician can refer you to a rheumatologist both to make or confirm the diagnosis and to suggest or initiate treatment.

Rheumatology is a relatively young specialty. Nevertheless, you can expect that a rheumatologist will have graduated from medical school, been trained in internal medicine for at least two years, then served a fellowship in rheumatology for two or three years in an accredited training program. Evidence of successful completion of such training is dual board certification in internal medicine and in rheumatology, generally by the American Board of Internal Medicine or the American Osteopathic Board of Internal Medicine.

Some physicians trained in foreign countries may have different qualifications and credentials. You can tell if your rheumatologist is board-certified by checking the ABIM web site (www.abim.org).

In the United States, approximately 4,000 rheumatologists are currently in active practice, but as with many other medical specialists, they are not evenly distributed throughout the country. They tend to concentrate in larger cities and in academic medical centers, although this is not universally true. Many practice in groups, either with other rheumatologists or in groups of other specialists, but many communities have no rheumatologists at all. If you live in such a community, frequent hands-on treatment by a rheumatologist is not practical. Fortunately, rheumatologists are trained to work with primary-care physicians, who can supervise and monitor treatment of properly diagnosed patients with care plans.

Treating Arthritis

Although arthritic diseases can seldom be cured, the good news is that there is treatment for all of them. Depending on the type and severity of the arthritis, this may run the gamut from mild physical and/or occupational therapy to aggressive medical and surgical therapy. As we consider the different types of arthritis in this book, we shall review the treatments available for each in some detail, putting them in the context of specific patients, with some attention to the side effects you might encounter.

Are There Medications to Treat Arthritis?

Depending on your type of arthritis, your doctor may prescribe any combination of the following medications:

- Anti-inflammatory agents, ranging from mild and familiar oral medications such as aspirin to powerful new medicines that must be given by injection, such as etanercept and infliximab

- Immunosuppressive medicines, which inhibit the immune system (used especially in advanced cases of rheumatoid arthritis)

- Antibiotics (often used in infectious arthritis cases)

- Uric acid–lowering agents (typically used to treat gout)

- Corticosteroids (cortisone-like drugs that are taken systemically or injected into the involved joints)

Generic drug names In many cases, after a drug's initial patent period expires (by law, 20 years after it is invented), different companies market the same drug under a variety of names. Which brand name would we then use? The same thing may happen when a drug previously requiring a prescription becomes available over the counter (OTC). As an example, ibuprofen by prescription is called Motrin, but the OTC forms include Advil, Nuprin, and Motrin-IB.

To add to the confusion, companies may market the same drug under different names in different countries; for instance, indomethacin is Indocin in the United States, but Indocid in many other countries. Moreover, discarded names of withdrawn drugs may be recycled and used for totally different drugs. The prescription painkiller zomepirac, known as Zomax initially, was withdrawn from the market more than two decades ago. The name Zomax now refers to one company's brand of azithromycin, a familiar antibiotic, marketed in the United States as Zithromax. I'd rather spare you from this kind of confusion, so I will refer to all drugs in this book by their generic names. Nevertheless, for the sake of convenience, appendix 2 lists the generic names of the drugs mentioned in the book, along with a selection of brand names current at the time of this writing.

Bringing drugs to market Since drugs play such an important role in the treatment of most forms of arthritis, it is worth considering, at least briefly, the processes by which these drugs are discovered or invented, tested, approved, and released for general use.

Until fairly recently, most drugs employed in the treatment of arthritis were already in existence for some other medical purpose Their antiarthritic effects were, for the most part, serendipitously discovered when the drugs were given for another reason to someone who happened to have arthritis, producing an unexpected beneficial effect on the arthritis. Gold salts, for example, were used to treat certain chronic infections such as tuberculosis. Antimalarial drugs were used to prevent or treat malaria. Methotrexate and other chemotherapy drugs were used to treat cancer. Most of these medicines came into widespread use in treating arthritis based on anecdotal experience—that is, without their having undergone rigorous investigation for either effectiveness or safety in arthritis patients. Doctors began using methotrexate to treat rheumatoid arthritis in the 1960s, but studies validating its use for this indication were not reported until 20 years later.

More recently, pharmaceutical companies have been making new drugs designed specifically for treating arthritis. These drugs are of two general types. The more common ones are the "me too" drugs, based on existing drugs but modified either to achieve greater convenience of administration (for example, once- or twice-a-day dosing rather than four times a day) or improved safety (for example, COX-2–inhibiting nonsteroidal anti-inflammatory drugs—NSAIDs for short—with improved gastrointestinal safety). The second type includes the truly innovative drugs, like the TNF-alpha inhibitors, which work by novel mechanisms such as blockade of a specific, recently identified inflammatory mediator, and are clearly more effective than their predecessors.

Both types of new drugs go through extensive prerelease testing for safety (phase 1) and effectiveness (phase 2), requiring an average of seven years from the time the drugs are developed. When the data are available, the U.S. Food and Drug Administration (FDA) reviews them and determines whether the new drug is effective and safe enough to be approved so that doctors can prescribe it. There is some urgency to this, because the patent clock starts ticking when the drug is developed, not at the time it is released by the FDA, and once the 20-year patent has expired, the drug goes into the public domain, where it can be manufactured and sold by anyone who can meet certain FDA standards. Thus the company that bore the entire risk and considerable cost associated with developing and testing the new drug no longer has exclusive rights to it.

Given these pressures, it becomes somewhat easier to understand how some relatively uncommon side effects of a new drug might not be recognized during the testing phases. When recognition of such side effects eventually does occur, there is often pressure to force the pharmaceutical company to withdraw the drug in question, sometimes accompanied by accusations of duplicitous suppression of negative data by the manufacturer (which, unfortunately, has occasionally turned out to be true).

Can My Arthritis Be Treated with Surgery?

Orthopedic surgeons can perform certain types of surgery to repair or reconstruct some damaged joints that are painful or causing disability because they are no longer mechanically functional. Progress in joint replacement technology applicable to large weight-bearing joints—hips and knees—has been dramatic over the past three decades, and highly satisfactory results are now commonplace. In some cases, shoulder or elbow replacement surgery can give good results as well. Wrist and ankle replacements are more problematic, but this technology is developing. Lesser procedures are also appropriate in some cases.

Can Physical or Occupational Therapy Help?

Physical and occupational therapy have an important place in the treatment of arthritis. Passive modalities, such as applying heat, and active strengthening and range-of-motion exercises also offer benefits to many patients. Because of the differing needs of patients with different forms of arthritis or in different stages of any form of arthritis, these therapy programs need to be individually designed and supervised by trained professionals. These include physiatrists (specialists in physical medicine and rehabilitation, not to be confused with psychiatrists), physical therapists, and occupational therapists.

A Word on Depression

As a chronic, unrelenting problem, arthritis also takes an emotional toll that can seriously tax a person's normal coping mechanisms. Patients suffering from arthritis frequently find themselves also suffering from depression—it isn't easy to be constantly in pain or even just persistently uncomfortable. Furthermore, depression can amplify pain. It can also be emotionally difficult to deal with a chronic illness that you can treat but not completely cure. If you have recently been diagnosed with arthritis or if you think you may have arthritis, and you are suffering from depression, please talk to your doctor. Some common signs of depression are sadness, loss of appetite and weight loss, unexplained tiredness, inability to concentrate, and inability to sleep. These signs are not specific for depression, however, and they require investigation to ascertain the cause.

Not everybody with arthritis needs to see a psychiatrist or a psychologist, but some do. Depression is a real illness that affects families—spouses and children—of patients. It puts stress on marriages, drains finances, and limits productivity. Marital and family counseling may also be a helpful component to your treatment plan.

Chapter 2

Rheumatoid Arthritis

Onset: The Nightmare Begins

Life was good for Beulah. She was an attractive 23-year-old executive secretary, happily married for one year, and she had just begun thinking about starting a family. Her husband, Clifford, three years older than she, was an engineer with an excellent future in the aerospace industry. They met at a college mixer, began dating, and then married right after they both graduated. They seemed to be the perfect couple: young, in love, and living the American dream, with their future bright before them. Then, without warning, their world began to collapse.

One day Clifford noticed a small lump in his neck. It wasn't sore, so he ignored it. But the lump didn't go away. When he realized that it was gradually getting bigger, he consulted his physician. The lump was an enlarged lymph node. After reviewing the biopsy (tissue specimen from the lymph node), his doctor diagnosed him with non-Hodgkin's lymphoma, an aggressive, malignant cancer of the lymphatic system.

Over the next few months, despite aggressive treatment, Clifford got sicker and sicker. His spleen and liver were affected. He lost 40 pounds. It was hard to tell which made him more miserable—the disease or the treatment. Soon it became clear that Clifford wasn't going to make it. Beulah was beside herself with worry. Although she tried to act brave around her husband, she was devastated emotionally and, to an increasing extent, physically.

Shortly after Clifford's diagnosis, Beulah began to feel stiff, particularly in her hands and wrists, and she noticed some puffiness in these regions.

Soon the symptoms spread to her shoulders, elbows, hips, knees, ankles, and feet. Even her jaw joints were painful, and her voice became hoarse.

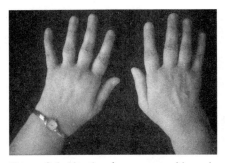

Figure 2-1: Hands of a person with early, as yet nondestructive, rheumatoid arthritis. The same joints are affected in both hands (symmetrical), and the distal joints of the fingers (most distant from the wrists) are usually spared.

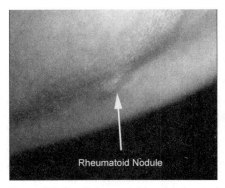

Rheumatoid Nodule

Figure 2-2: Small rheumatoid nodule located just below the elbow. This is a typical location, but nodules may be found in many other sites as well.

As Clifford progressively went downhill, so did Beulah, although she tried to conceal her discomfort when she was around him. But she had increasing difficulty carrying out simple tasks: opening jars, turning faucets on and off, and typing. She was taking large doses of aspirin, which gave her some relief but her stomach was rebelling. She was so focused on her husband's plight that she didn't take proper care of her own worsening problems.

Clifford died almost six months to the day after his diagnosis. By then Beulah was so disabled that she could hardly get through the wake and the funeral. She really became scared when she noticed some lumps under her skin, just below the elbows.

The lumps weren't sore, just as Clifford's first swollen lymph node had been pain-free. As soon as Clifford was buried, Beulah scheduled an appointment with her internist to find out what her

problem was. After an examination and some tests, he sat down with
her to discuss the findings.

Beulah's Assessment

Beulah's doctor immediately recognized the signs of rheumatoid
arthritis. Her story was fairly typical for the way the disease often
begins: onset of pain, stiffness, and swelling in many joints, especially
the small joints of the hands, wrists, and jaw (temporomandibular)
in a young woman, often preceded by a traumatic event.

The doctor was able to confirm the diagnosis by noting that the
distribution of the joints affected was mostly symmetrical and that
the lumps below Beulah's elbows were typical rheumatoid nodules:
firm, spherical, nontender masses of tissue under the skin, about a
half-inch in diameter. He also suspected that her hoarseness might be
caused by arthritis of the joints in the voice box (crico-arytenoid), a
fairly common occurrence with rheumatoid arthritis.

Beulah's blood tests showed mild anemia (low red blood
cell count), and additional lab tests for inflammatory activity—
sedimentation rate and C-reactive protein (CRP)—were elevated.
Both of these tests detect proteins in the blood whose concentration
is increased by the presence of inflammation in the body. Furthermore, the tests revealed an abnormal antibody in her blood called
a *rheumatoid factor.* This is an autoantibody directed against IgG,
a normal blood protein. Rheumatoid factor is present in about 4
in 5 people with rheumatoid arthritis, but it is also often found in
several other conditions, as well as in some older people without
any apparent disease.

• • • *Fast Fact* • • •

An antibody that reacts against components of your
own body is called an autoantibody.

• • •

Beulah's doctor referred her to a specialist in rheumatology, experienced in the diagnosis and treatment of arthritis.

What did the specialist say?

The rheumatologist reviewed the X-rays of Beulah's chest, hands, and wrists, noting that the films of the hands showed no erosions around the small joints typical of destructive rheumatoid arthritis. But there did appear to be some calcium loss in the bones adjacent to the joints. This was due to a condition called juxta-articular osteoporosis, which is often seen in early stages of the disease. He also observed that her wrists had similar calcium loss, but there were no erosions there either. This was good news. He concluded that despite her delay in seeking treatment, the rheumatoid arthritis had not yet caused a lot of destruction.

With regard to the chest X-ray, Beulah's specialist and internist were looking for several abnormalities, none of which, fortunately, was present. Sometimes an inflammatory form of arthritis is the earliest sign of cancer, especially lung cancer. Some people with true rheumatoid arthritis get rheumatoid nodules—like those Beulah had at her elbows—in the lungs, where they look very similar to cancer on an X-ray. Rheumatoid arthritis can be associated with other chest X-ray findings as well, including an accumulation of fluid around the lungs—known as pleural effusion—or fibrous changes in the lung tissue. A few people with tuberculosis and other uncommon infectious

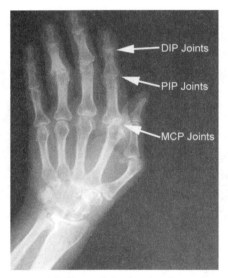

Figure 2-3: X-ray of the hands of a patient with destructive rheumatoid arthritis. Several of the PIP (proximal interphalangeal) and MCP (metacarpophalangeal) joints are damaged, but the DIP (distal interphalangeal) joints are spared.

diseases get arthritis as a symptom. As it turned out, Beulah's chest X-ray was clear.

Based on all this information, the rheumatologist agreed with the diagnosis of rheumatoid arthritis and began mapping out a course of treatment.

All about Rheumatoid Arthritis

What causes rheumatoid arthritis?
Did I "catch" this disease?

We don't know what causes rheumatoid arthritis, despite years of research. It's one of the autoimmune diseases, in the sense that immune mechanisms somehow become misdirected. Instead of protecting us from infections and malignancies, they attack components of our own bodies. These mechanisms cause inflammation in various tissues, most characteristically the tissues that line the joints, called the synovial membranes. This inflammation is ultimately destructive if it isn't controlled.

Among the suggested possible causes of rheumatoid arthritis is infection. Some infections are known to activate the immune system to cause autoimmune damage. An example is a particular strain of streptococcus, a common cause of sore throat that can lead to rheumatic fever or acute kidney disease by inducing self-destructive immune activity. Although great efforts have been expended to identify such a cause for rheumatoid arthritis, it hasn't been possible to do so. There's no convincing evidence that a person can "catch" rheumatoid arthritis from someone else.

Although the cause is unknown, some peculiar features of the disease are probably clues to its cause, if only we knew how to interpret them. For instance, there is evidence from the study of ancient human remains that rheumatoid arthritis appeared relatively recently in our history; there is no evidence that the disease existed among Europeans in the "Old World," (before 1500 CE) but Native American populations may have been affected earlier. Statements in the older medical literature to the effect that examinations of ancient Egyptian skeletons revealed evidence of rheumatoid arthritis have been superseded by the more recent recognition that the abnormalities seen there were due to ankylosing spondylitis, not rheumatoid arthritis. Rheumatoid arthritis is about three times more frequent in women than in men. There are two peaks in the age of onset, the first relatively early—15 to 35 years of age—and the other around age 70. For reasons we can't explain, the number of new diagnoses in the United States seems to be declining.

What was the role of the traumatic event—Clifford's illness and death?

The relationship between acute stress and immune function has been the subject of some investigation and a lot of speculation. Some studies have suggested that hormones originating in the nervous system—neurohormones, if you will—play an important role in regulating immune function. These systems can be disrupted by stress, whether emotional or physical. Many believe that such a mechanism may underlie the frequent observation that autoimmune diseases, especially rheumatoid arthritis, appear to be triggered or aggravated by stressors. The list of the top emotional stressors—first reported by U.S. Navy physicians Thomas Holmes and Richard Rahe in 1967, and now known as the Holmes-Rahe stress scale—is headed by death of a spouse.

How common is rheumatoid arthritis?

Roughly 1.3 million Americans suffer from rheumatoid arthritis, with about three times as many women as men.

Is rheumatoid arthritis genetic?

There does seem to be a genetic predisposition to rheumatoid arthritis, which is more common in people who have a family history of the disease. In particular, scientists have found an association between RA and a certain inherited blood cell antigen known as HLA (human leukocyte antigen)-DR4. An antigen is a substance that causes the body to make a specific immune response. This association acts as a susceptibility factor rather than a direct link to the cause of the disease, since many people with HLA-DR4 do not have rheumatoid arthritis. Any of the rheumatoid patient's children who inherit HLA-DR4 have an increased likelihood of getting the disease. That does not mean that they will surely develop rheumatoid arthritis or that children without the antigen won't, but it does increase the odds.

Rheumatoid arthritis and pregnancy

Rheumatoid arthritis itself is not known to interfere with fertility. However, many of the drugs used to treat it are potentially hazardous to the developing child during pregnancy, while others can make conception difficult or impossible, at least while they are being taken. Interestingly, pregnancy may have a beneficial effect on rheumatoid disease activity, possibly enabling some women patients to reduce the dosage of one or more of the drugs they take—maybe even to eliminate their medications entirely. Still, it's better not to become pregnant while on antirheumatic drug therapy.

Does rheumatoid arthritis predispose me to other diseases?

Rheumatoid arthritis is sometimes complicated by the simultaneous occurrence of other autoimmune diseases. Some relatively uncommon complications of rheumatoid arthritis include blood vessel inflammation (vasculitis) and eye inflammation (scleritis and scleromalacia). With modern drug treatment, we seldom encounter such problems these days.

There are, however, a few more common autoimmune diseases that rheumatoid arthritis patients must be alert to.

Sjögren's syndrome Sjögren's syndrome is named after famous Swedish eye surgeon Henrik Samuel Conrad Sjögren, who first recognized it in the early 1930s. In this condition, which occasionally occurs in people with rheumatoid arthritis, the eyes and mouth become very dry because the autoimmune response destroys the salivary glands and the tear glands. The disease may also attack endocrine glands such as the thyroid. In Sjögren's syndrome, the immune abnormality is often more profound than in rheumatoid arthritis alone, which leads to an increased incidence of certain malignancies, including especially lymphoma, multiple myeloma, and leukemia.

Carpal tunnel syndrome Carpal tunnel syndrome is fairly common and believed to be due to repetitive trauma, often affecting people who spend many hours a day working at a computer keyboard. But it can also be a complication of inflammation and swelling at the wrist in rheumatoid arthritis. In carpal tunnel syndrome, the median nerve—the main nerve that supplies the thumb, index finger, and part of the third finger—becomes entrapped and compressed at the wrist, leading to pain and tingling in these fingers, while sparing the ring finger and the fifth finger. If untreated, permanent damage to the nerve can result, leading to loss of muscle mass in the thenar eminence, the large muscle at the base of the thumb. Other nerve entrapment syndromes are less common, but they can also occur in rheumatoid arthritis.

Amyloidosis Amyloidosis is a term used to describe deposits of an unstructured, waxy, translucent substance in various organs. It's a complication of active rheumatoid arthritis and other chronic inflammatory diseases that remain uncontrolled over a long period. In some parts of the body, amyloidosis is nothing more than a nuisance, but in the kidneys or the muscles, especially the heart muscle, the condition can become life threatening by interfering with organ function. It's better to control the arthritis adequately up front, in the hope of avoiding amyloidosis, than to try treating it once it has occurred.

Can diet help?

We live in the age of organic nutrition and alternative therapies, and some people believe that proper nutrition can take care of almost any problem. However, this is a formula for disaster in rheumatoid arthritis. The only such treatment for which there is even a modicum of supportive data is the ingestion of fish oil because of its anti-inflammatory activity. Although large statistical studies show that arthritic patients on a diet high in fish oil do a little better than those on no special diet, the benefit is small and the amount of oil needed to achieve it is formidable, to say the least. In Europe and Australia, there are those who advocate gluten-free diets (gluten is a wheat protein), avoiding chocolate and red meat, and other dietary interventions, but little evidence of their efficacy exists.

The best dietary advice for a patient with arthritis is: don't get fat. Carrying around excess weight is a sure way to pulverize your arthritic knees. Eating moderately and exercising judiciously (using appropriate activities) are the keys to keeping your weight in check and thus helping to ease pain. Incidentally, starvation dieting won't work because the antirheumatic medications, many of which are rough on the GI tract, must be taken with food.

Should I exercise if I have rheumatoid arthritis?

One of the biggest problems for people with arthritis, whether it is rheumatoid or some other form, is that painful joints tend to make you less active. Who wants to run a mile when you ache with every step? However, avoiding exercise and physical activity in general begins a vicious cycle: the inactivity leads to muscle wasting, which in turn leads to decreased strength and even less activity, until a person becomes completely disabled. Inactivity also promotes weight gain, another big problem for all the obvious health reasons as well as the extra burden on arthritic, weight-bearing joints.

On the other hand, certain kinds of activity can be destructive to joints that may already have some damage from arthritis. Generally, if you are diagnosed with rheumatoid arthritis, you should avoid high-impact exercises such as running. Walking is a good alternative, and swimming is even better. It's important for you to follow an exercise program designed by a physical medicine expert, such as a physiatrist or a physical or occupational therapist, in order to minimize the likelihood of causing damage to joints and tendons.

Treating Rheumatoid Arthritis

Recent studies have shown that, left untreated, rheumatoid arthritis almost always produces disabling joint deformities. This has led to a change in the philosophy of treatment from the older conservative approach ("go low, go slow") to a much more aggressive early medical attack on the disease. There is some evidence that this can prevent some of the joint destruction, thus improving productivity and quality of life. The potential downside, however, is that this increases the risk of your experiencing treatment side effects.

The treatment of rheumatoid arthritis employs a number of potentially toxic drugs that need to be monitored closely. Drug toxicity is a big worry. The field has already seen the significant side effects of certain drugs that have been in use for many years, and there are concerns about the long-term hazards of the more recently introduced drugs. These latter drugs are increasingly used because of their outstanding effectiveness. It is critical that you take your medications exactly as prescribed and continue to visit your physician regularly for monitoring.

Can rheumatoid arthritis be managed successfully?

Yes. Your doctor and specialist can choose from a number of pharmaceutical and surgical options in customizing an effective treatment plan for you. If caught early, before permanent damage occurs, rheumatoid arthritis can be managed and contained. And with proper ongoing treatment, patients can live a relatively normal, pain-free life.

What factors are considered when choosing a treatment plan?

Beulah's doctor could have started with an antimalarial and an NSAID, planning to add methotrexate later if needed. Because of the time frame in which these drugs work, however, he would have had to wait at least two months before starting methotrexate. Based on the initial severity of Beulah's arthritis, he felt strongly that methotrexate would be needed, and he didn't want the disease to remain active for that length of time, during which it could inflict a lot of damage.

Methotrexate belongs to the category of DMARDs, which stands for disease-modifying antirheumatic drugs. These drugs can modify the course of rheumatoid arthritis in some patients, delaying and perhaps preventing erosion of the affected joints. Other DMARDs include injectable and oral gold, d-penicillamine, azathioprine, leflunomide, and sulfasalazine. Although these drugs are effective in some patients, they are typically more toxic and/ or less effective than methotrexate. Some can be used along with methotrexate in very severe cases. They are also usually slower to act than methotrexate. Beulah's rheumatologist explained that his strategy was to hold them in reserve in case she had an unacceptable response to the methotrexate (either a significant side effect or ineffectiveness).

He considered starting her on a low dose of prednisone, too. Prednisone is a synthetic cortisone-like drug that has been available for many years. It works fast and provides symptomatic relief, at least initially, for most patients. He ultimately decided against this as a first-line approach because of the drug's side effects over time, especially its tendency to cause osteoporosis, even in low doses. Once started, prednisone is very difficult to discontinue because it suppresses the body's ability to make its own cortisone.

Beulah's Treatment

Beulah's rheumatologist had some good news for her: modern medications have much to offer. Because she tested positive for rheumatoid factor (seropositive arthritis) and presented with rheumatoid nodules and multiple joint involvement—all indicators of potentially destructive disease—he recommended starting treatment with several medications.

Medication

As noted above, Beulah's doctor wanted to start with three basic medications:

- A nonsteroidal anti-inflammatory drug. NSAIDs (pronounced EN-seds) work by inhibiting cyclooxygenases (COXs), a group of enzymes important in the body's production of prostaglandins—an important class of mediators of inflammation. The doctor picked naproxen for several reasons. Beulah had no history of peptic ulcer disease, liver disease, or kidney disease. If she'd had ulcers, an alternative might have been celecoxib, the only selective COX-2 inhibitor still on the market. COX-2 inhibitors are designed not to irritate the stomach lining—one potential side effect of the nonselective NSAIDs. Unfortunately, the two other COX-2 inhibitors that had been approved by the FDA were later found to cause coronary artery disease in some patients;

they are no longer available in this country. In people not prone to ulcers, like Beulah, celecoxib has no advantage over the more common, nonselective NSAIDs. Naproxen also has the virtues of twice-a-day dosing, reasonable effectiveness, and relatively low cost. The doctor told her to take the drug with food so as not to unduly risk causing an ulcer. Naproxen usually reaches full effectiveness within about ten days, although it sometimes confers an immediate benefit.

- An antimalarial drug. The effectiveness of this class of drugs in rheumatoid arthritis was one of the circumstantial pieces of evidence that suggested an infectious cause for rheumatoid arthritis in the 1950s. Now everyone admits that the reason for antimalarials' effectiveness is not clear. Beulah's doctor chose hydroxychloroquine for this purpose, taken twice a day. He explained that this drug has several side effects, the most serious (though rarest) of which is blindness. That got her attention, and she questioned him sharply about hydroxychloroquine. He reassured her that she could take it safely for as long as necessary if she did not exceed the recommended daily dose and remembered to have her eyes examined annually by an ophthalmologist. He also told her that hydroxychloroquine would not reach full effectiveness for at least two months, possibly three.

- An antimetabolic medication. Although there are a couple of choices here, Beulah's doctor chose methotrexate, a chemotherapy drug that inhibits the body's utilization of the B vitamin folic acid. This vitamin is important in DNA synthesis, which lies at the heart of cell reproduction. Thus methotrexate preferentially inhibits replication of the most rapidly dividing cell populations, which in active rheumatoid arthritis are the cells in the inflamed areas. Although methotrexate has been prescribed by some physicians to treat rheumatoid arthritis since the early 1960s, its widespread use in this disease did not begin until the mid-1980s.

By then, the medical profession had become convinced that methotrexate was unique among chemotherapeutic drugs in that it did not materially increase the risk of developing cancer. Beulah's rheumatologist told her that methotrexate could be taken safely as long as it was monitored by blood counts and blood tests for liver function at about three-month intervals. He recommended a starting dose of three tablets weekly and noted that it would take 6 to 12 weeks for the drug to achieve full effectiveness.

Because the main drugs that will eventually control rheumatoid arthritis aren't effective for weeks to months, Beulah's doctor suggested that she might get some immediate relief from an injection of a corticosteroid medication. She agreed to this, and he gave her the injection at once.

Beulah's Response to Treatment

With some trepidation, Beulah consented to the proposed treatment, received her corticosteroid injection, and started the three oral drugs. By the next day, she felt almost normal. Her symptoms had miraculously cleared, as her doctor had predicted. This was the effect of the corticosteroid injection, but he had warned her that this would be temporary and that she needed to take her other medications in order to maintain the benefit.

A week or so later, Beulah noticed that her vision was blurry. The eye toxicity of the antimalarial drug immediately came to mind, and she called her doctor. He reassured her that this was not the serious retinal toxicity associated with hydrochloroquine but rather was related to the drug's tendency to relax the small muscles in the eye that focus the lens. This is normally a temporary effect and clears without the need to stop the drug, and that was the case with Beulah.

Over the next few weeks, some of her arthritic symptoms gradually recurred, but not as severely as before treatment. Beulah felt well enough to return to work, and as the weeks went by, and the long-acting drugs became effective, most of her symptoms again subsided. Her only problem was chronic mild inflammation in the right wrist, which eventually led to loss of motion in this joint. She followed the recommended testing regimen, including annual eye examinations and blood tests every three months, and had no further problems for the next couple of years.

Then one day Beulah began to have irregular vaginal bleeding. She consulted her gynecologist, who tried several approaches, including a dilatation and curettage (D and C), with no benefit. The gynecologist suspected that methotrexate might be the culprit and recommended that it be discontinued. With her rheumatologist's agreement, Beulah stopped methotrexate, and the bleeding subsided almost immediately.

Over the next few weeks, however, her arthritis became more active in multiple joints, especially the right wrist. After a second trial of methotrexate, which controlled the arthritis but again caused vaginal bleeding, it was clear that Beulah was not going to be able to use methotrexate.

What if a treatment stops working?

When a medication for rheumatoid arthritis loses its effectiveness or has to be discontinued because of side effects, several choices have to be made, depending on the circumstances. If the drug has lost its effectiveness, sometimes the solution is simply to increase the dose. There are limits to this approach, however, since the risk of side effects generally heightens as we increase the dose. Obviously, this was not the solution to Beulah's problem, as she already had experienced an intolerable side effect of methotrexate. The other option is to seek out a replacement for the current medication.

TNF-alpha inhibitors One possible alternative would have been another DMARD. However, since the onset of Beulah's illness, the FDA had approved a new class of apparently safe medications for rheumatoid arthritis: TNF-alpha inhibitors. These drugs block the action of a potent inflammatory mediator called tumor necrosis factor-alpha, or TNF-alpha, one of the inflammatory mediators collectively known as cytokines.

Nevertheless, enthusiasm for the use of TNF-alpha inhibitors was tempered by several facts. It was worrisome that nothing was known of the long-term toxicity of these agents, since they had been in use only since 1998. Furthermore, they could be administered only by injection. In addition, they were extremely expensive. Despite these drawbacks, Beulah's rheumatologist felt that a TNF-alpha inhibitor might be the best solution to her current dilemma. After testing her for latent tuberculosis with a skin test (which was negative), he began the application process with her insurance company to get preauthorization to start her on etanercept, the first of the TNF-alpha inhibitors approved for use in rheumatoid arthritis.

Beulah learned to inject herself with etanercept weekly, rotating among several injection sites, as she had been instructed. Within a few weeks, she felt normal for the first time since the onset of her arthritis. She was only slightly limited by the damage to her right wrist and continued to do well for several more years.

Other TNF-alpha inhibitors currently approved for treating rheumatoid arthritis are infliximab and adalimumab. All are quite effective. They differ somewhat in the route and frequency of administration, but all must be injected. Etanercept is a genetically engineered, synthetic receptor for TNF-alpha, while infliximab and adalimumab are monoclonal antibodies that bind TNF-alpha.

Other cytokine inhibitors Inhibitors of other cytokines may also be helpful in rheumatoid arthritis. Anakinra, for example, blocks interleukin-1 (IL-1), another cytokine important in inflammation. Anakinra's early record for safety has also been good. Abatacept blocks the cooperation among sets of certain cells required for inflammation. Rituximab, a monoclonal antibody that specifically attacks human antibody-producing cells, also has proven beneficial in some patients who do not respond adequately to other therapies. These new treatments, along with others that remain experimental, are products of recombinant DNA technology. It is likely that this technology will provide us with many additional new drugs over the next few years.

What are the side effects of these newer treatments?

Although the great majority of people tolerate TNF-alpha inhibitors quite well, some serious side effects have been seen in a few patients. Using these drugs can decrease your resistance to infection, sometimes with serious consequences. Unsuspected inactive (latent) tuberculosis can be activated, resulting in a rapid, life-threatening spread throughout the body. You can avoid this, however, by having a tuberculosis skin test before starting the drug. A few patients have developed a multiple sclerosis–like neurological disorder that can, in some cases, affect vision, as well as other neurological functions. Occasionally patients may also develop an autoimmune syndrome that resembles lupus erythematosus (see chapter 8 for a description of this disease). Obviously, if any of these problems appear, stop the drug immediately and inform your physician.

The newer drugs mentioned have not been around long enough for us to become aware of possible serious delayed side effects. This concern arises from the fact that many other powerful immunosuppressive drugs used to treat rheumatoid arthritis—mainly chemotherapeutic drugs originally designed to treat cancer—may cause cancer themselves, sometimes decades later. Historically, this tendency did not become apparent until 20 years or more after their introduction for this use. Examples of such drugs are azathioprine and cyclophosphamide. Methotrexate, on the other hand, has been used to treat rheumatoid arthritis for almost a half century, with no evidence that it causes cancer.

What to Expect

Will I be disabled?

Only time can truly answer this question. In some cases, the disease is mild and responds to minimal treatment. In others, it is hard to control and very aggressive, attacking not only the joints but many other tissues as well, including the small blood vessels, eyes, lungs, and heart. Most of the time, however, the disease smolders along relentlessly; unless it can be controlled, over time it can do a lot of damage to the joints.

Rheumatoid arthritis treatment improved dramatically during the last quarter of the twentieth century, and there is now evidence that some medications can slow or prevent joint damage in many people, assuming that they can tolerate the medications. Medications can't reverse damage that has already occurred, but today's surgical reconstructive procedures offer much more hope than in the past.

Beulah's Outcome

As of this writing, Beulah has had rheumatoid arthritis for 12 years. Although she is doing well, the disease has caused some permanent damage to her right wrist, and the potential for more damage exists. Her body has rejected one effective treatment (methotrexate), and it may reject others. And unknown long-term side effects of her medications may yet emerge.

Beulah may eventually need surgery to reconstruct her damaged joints. Wrist replacement surgery has not yet come of age, but very good options exist for the hips, knees, shoulders, and elbows.

Disease at a Glance:
Rheumatoid Arthritis

Who Gets It?

- Most frequent onset in women of childbearing age
- Weak heredity component (no specific gene identified)
- 1.3 million Americans affected

Joint Involvement

- Generally involves multiple joints
- Affects same joints on both sides of the body
- Erodes and destroys joint tissues

Other Features and Complications

- Rheumatoid nodules
- Vasculitis
- Sjögren's syndrome
- Scleritis and scleromalacia
- Amyloidosis

Lab Results

- Rheumatoid factor in 80 percent of patients
- Elevated sedimentation rate and C-reactive protein

Treatment

- General
  - Adequate rest
  - Appropriate exercise
  - Education
- Medications
  - Aspirin or other NSAID
  - Antimalarial drug
  - Methotrexate and/or other DMARD
  - TNF-alpha inhibitor or other biological agent
  - Local joint injections
- Surgery if appropriate

Although Beulah's course can be viewed as an example of how things may go in rheumatoid arthritis, every patient is different. There are few clues that allow us to predict how an individual patient will respond to any treatment. For example, Beulah's menstrual abnormalities are an unusual complication of methotrexate, but she hasn't had any of the more common complications: liver function abnormalities, suppression of blood cell production, nausea, hair loss, and inflammation of the lungs

Beulah is what we doctors refer to as a "good" patient. She is bright and communicative, and participates thoughtfully in her own care. She makes an effort to listen to her body and to learn the potentials and limitations of her treatment. She has a good sense of humor and supportive people around. All of these characteristics work to her benefit and will help to ensure the best outcome possible.

Chapter 3

Osteoarthritis

Onset: I Must Be Getting Old!

It was the first morning of Harry's retirement. For almost everybody else, Monday was a workday, but not for Harry. Not any longer. He luxuriated in sleeping in, which for him meant not getting up until six-thirty. He was looking forward to working in the yard that day. It looked as though the weather would cooperate: the sun was out, and the birds were singing. Through the open window, he could hear the dull roar of the interstate a mile or so away and somewhat wistfully pictured himself on the road to the office, but he soon put that out of his mind and refocused his attention on getting out of bed and getting dressed.

Stella, Harry's wife, was already up and puttering around in the kitchen. Although she might have been a little jittery about having him home all the time, Harry was determined not to be a pest. No, he would just have his breakfast, especially the two cups of black coffee he always drank, read the paper, and start mowing the grass, a job he had "outsourced" for the last ten years.

As Harry headed for the shower, the stiffness that had been minimally bothering him for a few minutes each morning for the last several months began to clear, and the accustomed ache in his left groin began to improve as well. The shower and shave revived him further, and by the time he strolled into the kitchen in his jeans and work shirt, he was cheerful and ready for action.

At the breakfast table, Harry noticed that Stella seemed particularly grumpy. His wife wasn't a morning person, but this was a little unusual, even for her. It turned out that she too was suffering from joint pain—in her knees, which were also swollen, and her hands. When Harry confessed his own morning aches and discomfort, they agreed that they should visit the doctor together to "kill two birds with one stone."

On the way to the doctor's office, Stella revealed that she had been suffering with joint pain for years. "But it's just arthritis. Nothing anyone can do about it," she said dismissively. Her tendency toward stoicism had led her to just take a few aspirin and keep going without complaint, sure in the knowledge that joint paint was just a fact of life, something that came with advancing age.

Stella and Harry's Assessment

Soon after they arrived at the doctor's office, their physician questioned and examined both of them and ordered some blood tests and X-rays. Before they went to have these studies performed, however, he told them that he believed they both probably had osteoarthritis, and that Stella might be a candidate for surgery on her knee.

Stella, now age 60, had begun to notice intermittent aching in the right knee about five years previously. Until then, the knee hadn't bothered her since she twisted it taking a spill on the ice in her mid-twenties. It had swollen up then for a few days, but the swelling had gone down completely, leaving her with no symptoms except occasional clicking of the knee when she stretched it out after a period of inactivity. By the time she was 57, the right knee was always painful when she shifted her weight to that leg. Lately she had begun to notice recurrent swelling of the knee, worse at some times than at others, but always present. In addition, the knee felt unstable, and when she looked in the mirror, she noticed that her right leg was developing a knock-kneed appearance. The doctor told her that this was called a valgus deformity, that it was common in osteoarthritis of the knee, and that it was often, as in Stella's case, accompanied by joint instability, with a tendency for the knee to give way.

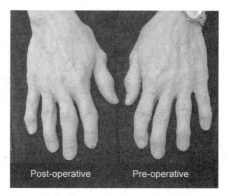

Post-operative   Pre-operative

For both Stella and Harry, X-ray confirmed the diagnosis of osteoarthritis. Stella had almost no cartilage left in the lateral compartment of her right knee, resulting in the knock-kneed appearance and the joint instability.

Although Stella had no X-rays taken of her hands, the doctor told her that they were arthritic as well. Based on the X-ray evidence, Harry had lost significant cartilage at the upper part of the left hip, making the joint space appear narrow as compared with the other side. And although he didn't know it, Harry's recurring groin pain was characteristic of osteoarthritis of the hip. The doctor told him that his left leg measured a little shorter than the right, and that the left hip's range of motion was somewhat restricted as compared with the right.

Figure 3-1: Bony enlargements at the DIP (distal interphalangeal) joints of a patient with osteoarthritis are called Heberden's nodes. In some patients, such enlargements are present at the PIP (proximal interphalangeal) joints, where they are called Bouchard's nodes. The Heberden's nodes on the right hand (shown on left) have been surgically removed, while those on the other hand are still present. Surgical removal of these enlargements is usually not necessary.

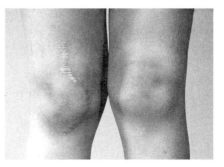

Blood tests were normal for both Stella and Harry, as is generally the case in osteoarthritis.

Figure 3-2: Knock-kneed (valgus) deformity, characteristic of osteoarthritis with loss of cartilage in the lateral compartments (outer sides) of the knees.

All about Osteoarthritis

What causes osteoarthritis?

As with most forms of arthritis, the exact cause of osteoarthritis is unknown. Unlike rheumatoid arthritis, which is an inflammatory condition of the joint membrane, or synovium, osteoarthritis is a degenerative condition of the joint cartilage, the shock-absorbing smooth cushion of gristle found in all normal joints. Inflammation does occur, but in osteoarthritis it is secondary to the mechanical irritation of the degenerated joint. Because an osteoarthritic joint is not necessarily inflamed, the name is something of a misnomer. The British call it osteoarthr*osis* to indicate that it is not basically an inflammatory condition.

Whatever the cause, most theories include some mechanical component of "wear and tear with inadequate repair" that appears to play a much greater role in osteoarthritis than in other arthritic conditions. The irritation produced by wear and tear causes abnormally robust bone growth locally, which is called hypertrophy and results in bony spurs forming around osteoarthritic joints.

Here are some factors that predispose a person to osteoarthritis.

Age Advancing age is one factor. Scientists think that the joint cartilage may contain less fluid in older men and women and therefore may become brittle and develop tiny cracks, leading the cartilage to deteriorate.

Previous injury Another possible factor is previous injury or damage to a joint, even injury caused by a disease like rheumatoid arthritis, which can have secondary osteoarthritis superimposed upon it. For example, it's possible that Stella's knee injury many years before may have produced a minimal degree of damage to the knee cartilage, and this ultimately brought about the osteoarthritis, especially since she didn't have it to the same degree in the opposite knee. A variation on this theme might be the late osteoarthritis that frequently develops in people with a history of congenital joint abnormalities, such as a dysplastic (deformed) or dislocated hip at birth.

Weight Obesity is another predisposing factor, particularly for weight-bearing joints like the hip and knee. Although both are large joints, studies have shown that the actual weight-bearing surface within them is small; perhaps no more than one square inch. Furthermore, the effective weight borne by this small area is multiplied many times by movement, especially running and jumping. These activities can impose tons of pressure within the joints, and this is magnified exponentially by increased body weight. So keeping your weight down can significantly protect the cartilage in your weight-bearing joints.

What are the symptoms of osteoarthritis?

At 60 years of age, Stella had always enjoyed good health, though she really did not make much of an effort to take care of herself. She was 15 pounds overweight and did not exercise (not counting her working incessantly around the house). When she was about 50, she began to notice that the outermost (distal) joints of her fingers were deformed, just like her mother and older sister.

These bony bumps were red and tender when they first appeared, but the inflammation gradually subsided. Although her

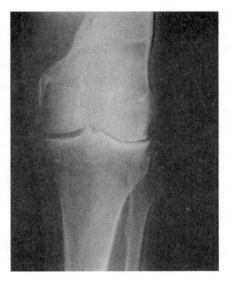

Figure 3-3: X-ray showing loss of joint "space" (actually cartilage) in the lateral compartment of the left knee in a patient with advanced osteoarthritis. The joint cartilage in the medial compartment (inner side) is reasonably well preserved.

finger joints ached when the weather was cold and wet, mostly the nodes were just unsightly and not much of an impediment.

Harry's health had also been good throughout his life. Unlike Stella, he took some pride in looking after himself. He was careful about what he ate, and he exercised regularly on a treadmill, even though it aggravated the pain in his left groin. Though he had regular physical examinations, he'd never complained about the discomfort there, which had troubled him every morning for months. He hadn't given much thought to his aches, especially since they occurred while he was busy getting ready for work every morning.

Is osteoarthritis genetic?

At least some forms of osteoarthritis appear to have a hereditary component. Heredity is particularly strong in osteoarthritis of the small joints of the hands, which varies in severity from mild to severe and is more frequent in women. Furthermore, congenital deformities of the hip joint—hip dysplasia—tend to run in families, and they often lead to secondary osteoarthritis.

There's also a rare, familial form of generalized osteoarthritis associated with tall stature and a spinal defect called spondyloepiphyseal dysplasia, which has been linked to a specific gene mutation. At least three families with this condition have been identified. The point of mentioning this is not to imply that most cases of osteoarthritis have a genetic component, but rather to illustrate that the condition can be inherited, perhaps in more cases than we know.

Red Flag

One of the most common symptoms of osteoarthritis of the hip is groin pain. Lateral hip pain or buttock pain does not usually originate in the hip joint itself, so many people misinterpret this early warning sign.

Can osteoarthritis be prevented?

Given the current lack of understanding of the mechanisms involved, the answer for now is probably not, but a lot of ongoing research hopes to change that. One fascinating approach is to find ways to speed up the cartilage repair process. A group of hormone-like chemicals called cytokines, secreted locally in joints, influences cartilage maintenance, suggesting that it may be possible to promote cartilage repair using one or some combination of these chemicals. Although no such treatment is ready for investigation in humans as yet, the concept is promising.

Can diet help?

A more mundane approach might be to reduce the wear and tear by maintaining your appropriate body weight and minimizing activities that are thought to damage cartilage, including stair climbing, carrying of heavy items, and high-impact actions like jumping and running. The role of diet beyond appropriate weight maintenance is controversial. For example, vitamin C, once believed to help protect against joint degeneration through strengthening connective tissue, now appears to actually increase the severity of osteoarthritis of the knees at high doses of more than 500 milligrams daily.

Another avenue might be to supply the body with the building blocks of cartilage. That is the theory behind the use of such so-called natural dietary supplements as glucosamine and chondroitin sulfate, which are biochemicals important in the structure of cartilage and other connective tissue. Although there is little evidence that taking these substances by mouth has any benefit in maintaining cartilage, they do ease pain for some people with osteoarthritis, and they appear to be safe. A recently published Italian study suggests that glucosamine may actually slow the progression of osteoarthritis of the knees.

Clearly, further study of the effects of diet and supplements on osteoarthritis is needed before we can determine the value of this approach.

Should I exercise if I have osteoarthritis?

Low-impact, non–weight-bearing exercises such as stretching, isometric strengthening, and range of motion are helpful for maintaining muscle strength and flexibility and are not harmful to the joint cartilage. Swimming is an ideal exercise for cardiovascular fitness in people with osteoarthritis.

How common is osteoarthritis?

According to the Arthritis Foundation, osteoarthritis affects almost 27 million Americans, mostly over 45 years of age, and is responsible for at least 7 million physician visits annually. Based on this information, it would certainly not be unusual for both members of a married couple in their sixties to have significant osteoarthritis. Furthermore, the Arthritis Foundation estimates that almost half of these men and women do not know what type of arthritis they have and, therefore, are not in a position to make informed decisions about treatment.

Why is osteoarthritis more common in women?

The short answer is that we don't really know. It is a fact, however, that most forms of arthritis, including osteoarthritis, are more common and tend to be more severe in women. Exceptions to this are the so-called seronegative spondyloarthropathies (see chapter 5), which tend to be more severe in men. Women are especially disproportionately afflicted by osteoarthritis of the fingers. The nodular deformities seen in osteoarthritic fingers are named according to their location: those of the outermost, or distal interphalangeal, joints are called Heberden's nodes, and those of the middle, or proximal interphalangeal, joints are called Bouchard's nodes. A recently described variant gene known as FRZB is associated with an increased risk of osteoarthritis of the hip in women; this variant gene interferes with bone and cartilage development.

Is there a relationship between osteoarthritis and osteoporosis?

There's probably not a direct link between osteoarthritis and osteoporosis, although the two conditions frequently occur together. In osteoporosis, bones lose calcium, so that people with this disorder are more likely to sustain fractures than they would otherwise. It's possible that the frequency with which the two conditions occur together relates to the facts that both are more common in women and both become more frequent as people get older.

Interestingly, osteoarthritis in the spine may mask the presence of osteoporosis. The test for bone density measures resistance by bone tissue to a measured dose of X-rays. If the bone density is low (due to low calcium content of bone, as in osteoporosis), this resistance is decreased, and higher than normal amounts of X-rays pass through. But low bone density may not be detectable by this method if bone mass is increased due to the bony hypertrophy, or overgrowth, associated with osteoarthritis of the spine. That's why measuring the bone density of the hip rather than the spine is a better way of assessing a person for generalized osteoporosis.

Treating Osteoarthritis

Can osteoarthritis be cured?

Just as it's currently not possible to prevent osteoarthritis, it's also not possible to cure it. Nevertheless, many avenues of treatment are available. They fall generally into four categories, as noted in chapter 1: (1) medications injected directly into the joint; (2) oral medications, which treat the problem systemically; (3) surgery; and (4) physical therapy.

Does osteoarthritis treatment predispose me to other diseases?

The treatments for osteoarthritis are not known to predispose patients to other diseases.

What factors are considered when choosing a treatment plan?

Since nonsteroidal anti-inflammatory medications (see below) play an important role in treatment, it is essential that you inform your doctor of any preexisting conditions that might be aggravated by these drugs. Examples include a history of peptic ulcer disease or gastritis, impaired kidney function due to any cause, the use of incompatible medications (for example, anticoagulants used to prevent abnormal formation of blood clots leading to heart attacks or strokes), bronchial asthma, or a history of allergy to NSAIDs. Moreover, some of the drugs (indomethacin, for instance) have an unfortunate tendency to cause depression or other mental disorders in elderly patients.

Surgery may be a part of the treatment plan; if a person's health is good otherwise, this generally would not present a problem, even if the patient is elderly. Preexisting heart disease or stroke would increase the risk of surgery. If a person is taking anticoagulants, these would generally need to be stopped prior to any type of surgery.

Stella's Treatment

Stella's doctor recommended that she consider knee surgery because the cartilage was almost gone in the lateral compartment, bringing about pain, inflammation, a "bone-on-bone" situation on X-ray (caused by the wearing away of cartilage that occurs in advanced osteoarthritis), and marked deformity and instability. He pointed out that oral medication probably would not provide adequate symptomatic relief, would not lead to cartilage repair, and would require high doses to get any benefit at all. Knee replacement surgery, on the other hand, would relieve Stella's pain and stabilize the joint.

Surgery

The doctor discussed with Stella the mechanics of knee replacement:

- She would need to see an orthopedic surgeon who subspecializes in adult reconstructive joint surgery. Some surgeons even subsubspecialize in a particular joint, such as the shoulder, knee, or hip.

- Once the surgeon agreed that total knee replacement (TKR) surgery was indicated, Stella would need a general physical examination to clear her for surgery, making sure that she didn't have any hidden problems that might increase the danger of the procedure—such as a partial blockage of the main arteries of the neck or the coronary arteries that supply the heart. Then the surgeon would schedule a date for the procedure.

- At some point in the process, the surgeon would discuss the various joint-replacement options: cemented versus uncemented (porous-surface) implants, various replacement materials and their costs versus expected useful life, and other matters on which she would make a decision.

- The surgeon would also discuss with Stella the expected recovery period and the rehabilitation protocol she would need after surgery, so that she would have a reasonably good idea of what to expect.

- When she understood all this, she would be asked to give her informed consent to have the procedure done.

Harry's Treatment

X-rays showed only moderate loss of cartilage in Harry's hip joint. The doctor determined that, for the short term at least, medications, exercises, and joint protection (avoidance of potentially damaging activities, as previously mentioned) might be sufficient. Other than osteoarthritis, Harry's health was good, and he had no other conditions that would make the use of anti-inflammatory medications especially risky.

Medication

Nonsteroidal (not cortisone-like) anti-inflammatory drugs—NSAIDs for short—provide moderately effective relief of symptoms caused by inflammation, including pain, redness, heat, and swelling. In some people, they produce excellent relief. These drugs work by inhibiting the cyclooxygenase (COX) group of enzymes, which are responsible for the production of inflammatory chemicals called prostaglandins. Examples of NSAIDs include aspirin, indomethacin, ibuprofen, naproxen, and many others.

Over the years, the pharmaceutical industry has brought many such drugs to the marketplace, citing improvements such as longer duration of action and/or lower risk of toxicity to justify patients' switching to the latest drug. Some of these medications proved so unexpectedly toxic—despite having passed FDA scrutiny for approval—that they later had to be taken off the market. Famous examples include benoxyprofen (Oraflex) and zomepirac (Zomax), in the early 1980s. Others, such as phenylbutazone (Butazolidin) and oxyphenbutazone (Tandearil), were always known to have frequent, serious side effects (including suppression of blood cell formation), and were removed when less dangerous alternatives became available.

Beginning in the late 1990s, a new class of NSAIDs, the COX-2 inhibitors, the prototypes of which are celecoxib, rofecoxib, and valdecoxib, became available. Rofecoxib, sold under the brand name Vioxx, had to be withdrawn from the market in September 2004 because a large study showed that it predisposed people to heart attacks. Valdecoxib (Bextra) followed suit in April 2005. There is also some data indicating that celecoxib may have the same problem, though perhaps not as severe. Because these drugs selectively inhibit only COX-2, they should theoretically be less likely to cause gastrointestinal bleeding. The jury is still out on whether celecoxib adds sufficient value to warrant its significantly higher cost and greater risk of side effects. Since rofecoxib and valdecoxib have been discontinued, celecoxib is the only COX-2 inhibitor available in the United States at this time.

Harry's doctor recommended that he try one of the nonselective NSAIDs. He wrote a prescription for 75 milligrams of diclofenac twice daily with food and warned Harry to watch for any new symptoms after starting this drug (or any other NSAID), particularly black, tarry stools, which might indicate gastrointestinal bleeding occurring soon after starting the drug or after prolonged use. He recommended that while taking the drug, Harry should have certain blood tests conducted at about six-month intervals, especially blood counts and serum creatinine levels, to detect evidence of blood loss and impaired kidney function, respectively.

Other treatments

The doctor also discussed with Harry the importance of keeping his body weight down, not carrying excessively heavy objects, and avoiding unnecessary stair climbing. He also suggested that for cardiovascular fitness, Harry should consider swimming three times a week for at least 30 minutes as his exercise of choice, since that activity, while exercising all muscle groups, is not weight-bearing. He reiterated how important it was to avoid or limit any activities that produce pain lasting more than two hours.

What other medications are there for osteoarthritis?

Earlier we considered some of the anti-inflammatory drugs available for managing osteoarthritis. But when doctors select and recommend these medications, they have a much larger list from which to choose than the medications we have looked at so far.

Nonsteroidal anti-inflammatory drugs (NSAIDs) The nonselective NSAIDs that to varying degrees inhibit both COX-1 and COX-2 have been introduced over the past three decades. Then there's aspirin, which has been around for nearly a century. The list of drug candidates is even longer in many foreign countries. Why are there so many drugs that do almost the same thing? Would patients be any worse off if there were only one or two such drugs?

Bringing a new NSAID to market is a time-consuming and costly process, but some new members of this category have been helpful to patients. For example, the early NSAIDs, like indomethacin and ibuprofen, are short-acting medications, which makes it necessary to take multiple doses daily to feel better. Some newer drugs, like naproxen, sulindac, and diclofenac, were designed for sustained relief, so that they might need to be taken only twice a day. Piroxicam was the prototype of long-acting NSAIDs that could be taken once daily, and nabumetone, too, provided a somewhat safer once-a-day alternative.

NSAID side effects Although all the nonselective NSAIDs have about the same toxicity profile across populations of users, the degree to which the different drugs produce various side effects varies from person to person. All the drugs have side effects in the liver, kidneys, gastrointestinal lining, bone marrow, central nervous system, and inner ear, but many people take them without suffering any of these effects, while others have one or more side effects with one drug but not another.

Here are the nonselective NSAIDs currently available in the United States, listed alphabetically according to their generic names, followed by common brand names in parentheses (also see appendix 2):

- acetylsalicylic acid (aspirin, Ascriptin, Bufferin)
- choline magnesium trisalicylate (Trilisate)
- diclofenac (Arthrotec, Cataflam, Solaraze, Voltaren)
- diflunisal (Dolobid)
- etodolac (Lodine)
- fenoprofen (Nalfon)
- flurbiprofen (Ansaid)
- ibuprofen (Advil, Motrin, Nuprin)
- indomethacin (Indocin)
- ketoprofen (Orudis, Oruvail)
- meclofenamate (Meclomen)
- meloxicam (Mobic)
- nabumetone (Relafen)
- naproxen (Aleve, Anaprox, Naprosyn)
- piroxicam (Feldene)
- salsalate (Disalcid, Salflex)
- sulindac (Clinoril)
- tolmetin (Tolectin)

Selective COX-2 inhibitors As noted above, there is a more recent subset of the NSAIDs that selectively inhibits COX-2 without inhibiting COX-1. Prostaglandins produced under the influence of COX-1 have a protective effect on the lining of the lower esophagus, the stomach, and the upper portion of the small intestine (duodenum). Therefore, the rationale behind the use of the selective COX-2 inhibitor celecoxib is to reduce the likelihood of NSAID-induced ulcers in the gastrointestinal tract. Although this benefit is not absolute, celecoxib seems to be better tolerated than the nonselective NSAIDs by people prone to peptic ulcer disease. The trade-off appears to be a somewhat greater risk of coronary artery disease. Furthermore, celecoxib is significantly more expensive than its nonselective counterparts. Applications for FDA approval of two additional COX-2 inhibitors (etoricoxib and lumiracoxib) are pending as of this writing, but considering the problems with their predecessors, prospects for their release seem dubious.

Other oral medications Acetaminophen (also spelled acetamenophen, known as paracetamol in the United Kingdom and Europe, and marketed in the United States as Tylenol) is a familiar pain reliever often used in osteoarthritis. This drug does not inhibit COX-1 or COX-2 and is not strongly anti-inflammatory. It does reduce the level of the recently discovered cyclooxygenase designated COX-3. This enzyme facilitates prostaglandin production in the central nervous system. The effectiveness of acetaminophen in osteoarthritis is, according to most observers, less than that of the more classical NSAIDs, but some people get significant pain relief from it. In large amounts, acetaminophen is toxic to the liver.

Glucosamine, often combined with chondroitin sulfate, is another pain reliever widely used in osteoarthritis. These chemicals are components of cartilage. Technically, they are not even really drugs; rather, the FDA classifies them as supplements, not subject to the same standards the FDA applies to drugs. The rationale behind the use of these agents is that since cartilage deterioration seems to be the basic lesion in osteoarthritis, replenishing some of cartilage's building blocks might be beneficial. Whether or not that is true, there is evidence that taking glucosamine and chondroitin sulfate provides some pain relief for some people. It is thought to be safe, with a few exceptions, to take these preparations, which are regulated not as drugs but rather as supplements by the FDA. People allergic to shellfish should avoid these preparations, because they are extracted from shellfish.

Injectable drugs When an osteoarthritic joint, such as a knee, becomes acutely inflamed, it may be beneficial for the physician to inject anti-inflammatory medication directly into the joint. This can provide rapid relief of pain and swelling, lasting for variable periods, sometimes up to several months. A corticosteroid preparation is the most common category of medication for injection into an osteoarthritic joint. These agents are analogs of hydrocortisone, and several long- and short-acting forms are available. They are usually injected along with a local anesthetic such as lidocaine to give more immediate relief than the corticosteroid alone.

Depending on which joint is to be injected, the procedure may be carried out with you sitting or lying down. In order to minimize the risk of introducing an infection, the physician cleanses the skin over the joint carefully with an antiseptic, often an iodine-containing solution followed by alcohol. After that, he may anesthetize the skin with lidocaine, injected through a small needle, or have an assistant "freeze" the skin with ethyl chloride spray. If necessary, joint fluid is removed for laboratory examination at this time. The corticosteroid injection is then administered. The whole procedure should take no more than five or ten minutes and should produce no more than minimal, temporary discomfort.

Hyaluronan, one of the main components of normal joint fluid, is an alternative medication for injection into osteoarthritic knees. This viscous lubricating material sometimes produces dramatic symptomatic relief. The usual routine is a series of three injections separated by one-week intervals. Although hyaluronan is expensive, some feel that it is a more physiological approach to osteoarthritis of the knee than corticosteroid injections since it chemically resembles normal joint fluid.

Stella and Harry's Response to Treatment

About four months after Stella and Harry first saw the doctor, Stella had a right total knee replacement. The orthopedic surgeon recommended that she have an uncemented porous-surface implant,

---

Disease at a Glance: Osteoarthritis

Who Gets It?
- 27 million Americans
- People over age 45
- More women than men
- A role for heredity in hand disease

Joint Involvement
- May affect one or more joints on one or both sides of the body
- Causes cartilage to thin, plus the formation of bone spurs and bone overgrowth

Lab Results
- Normal acute-phase reactants
- Negative blood test for rheumatoid factor

Treatment
- General
  — Adequate rest
  — Appropriate exercise
  — Education
- Medications
  — Aspirin or other NSAID
  — Local joint injections of corticosteroids or synthetic joint fluid
- Surgery if appropriate

which would be secured by ingrowth of bone rather than cement. She required about six weeks of postoperative rehabilitation, including muscle-strengthening exercises, and she gradually recovered. Stella's new knee was painless, stable, and much improved in appearance. The scar, which was pretty angry-looking initially, gradually improved in appearance as well.

Harry, meanwhile, started taking diclofenac. He made the suggested modifications to his activities and actually lost five pounds through careful attention to his diet and swimming regularly. His hip pain improved, but it never went away completely. He had no trouble with the medication and was able to continue taking it for many years.

What to Expect

Will I be disabled?

Given today's array of effective treatments, both medical and surgical, most people can get quality relief from the symptoms of osteoarthritis. Unless you have a number of preexisting health conditions that would rule out medications and surgery, it is unlikely that any severe disability could not be corrected.

Stella and Harry's Outcome

Stella's hands remained gnarled with osteoarthritis, but they didn't hurt and they functioned pretty well. The Heberden's and Bouchard's nodes were initially red and painful, but they responded to diclofenac and local heat, and the inflammation gradually went away. She was able to stop the drugs without her pain recurring or apparent further progression of the deformities.

A year or so after Harry's diagnosis at age 65, his right knee swelled up. The doctor thought it might be a result of unconsciously shifting his weight to the right because of the left hip problem.

A knee X-ray revealed minor osteoarthritis, so Harry's physician injected the joint with a corticosteroid preparation and cleared up the problem. Nevertheless, he told Harry that the relief was temporary and that the swelling would probably return. At age 75, Harry had a left total hip replacement with a good result—excellent pain relief and improved hip range of motion.

And they lived happily ever after.

Chapter 4

Gout

Onset: The Pitchfork from Hell

When the alarm went off at six in the morning, Elmer struggled to consciousness only to confront a pounding headache. He had been out on the town the night before with some buddies, celebrating the conclusion of a fat contract that would pave the way for his PR agency to add at least six more employees and move to plush quarters in the high-rent district. Along the way, he had imbibed liberal amounts of wine, and he was seriously hung over. Although he knew from previous experience that his current debilitated state would pass, he was pretty miserable at the moment. But he hadn't seen anything yet.

To say that Elmer swung his legs over the edge of the bed and hopped out would be a gross mischaracterization of the painstakingly careful, lumbering movements that followed, and it was several minutes before he felt capable of standing up. When he did finally attempt to stand, his entire consciousness was suddenly seized by a sensation that could only be likened to a red-hot nail's piercing the base of his right big toe. That pain, completely focused on a minuscule part of his more than ample body, squeezed out all other awareness. His headache was gone. Nothing mattered but the painful left big toe.

Upon examination, Elmer saw that his foot was swollen and had taken on a purplish hue around the base of the big toe. He tried gently rubbing the painful area but quickly thought better of it after setting off further jolts of pain.

Elmer immediately called his doctor, who suggested that he see a rheumatologist colleague. Elmer readily agreed. "Anything to get some relief!"

Elmer's Assessment

Despite bolts of pain, Elmer hobbled into the examining room, unwrapped his throbbing foot (he had not been able to get a shoe on it), and waited. In a few minutes, the doctor arrived, gingerly examined the right foot, asked Elmer a few questions, took his temperature, and performed a brief physical examination, focusing on Elmer's skin, particularly around the ears. Then he said, "Well, Elmer, it looks to me like you're having an attack of gout."

Acute inflammation in a single joint is called monoarticular arthritis, and the list of conditions that cause this is fairly short, with gout ranking at the top. The other main cause of monoarticular arthritis is infection. Although many different infectious agents, including bacteria, funguses, and viruses, can grow in a joint and cause arthritis, generally only bacterial infections tend to cause the acute and severe pain, heat, and swelling that Elmer was experiencing. Infectious agents can get into a joint by two main routes:

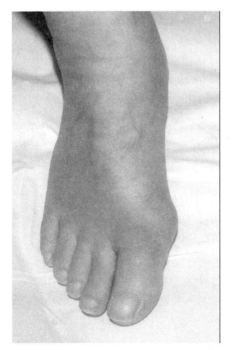

Figure 4-1: An acute attack of gout in the right big toe. It looks less impressive than it feels (just ask Elmer!).

via the bloodstream, or through a break in the skin. Staphylococcus and streptococcus are the most common agents that infect joints, but gonococcus, the cause of the sexually transmitted disease gonorrhea, is also noted for this.

Elmer had no fever, which increased the odds that his problem was gout rather than infection. However, fever is not a reliable differentiator of these two conditions.

Occasionally an injury, especially with a fracture, can mimic acute monoarticular arthritis. Elmer couldn't remember injuring the foot, but given his condition the night before, he could not rule it out either. The doctor suggested taking an X-ray in order to eliminate the possibility of a fracture but cautioned that a sprain wouldn't show up using this method. Furthermore, the films would usually still be normal so soon after the symptoms of either gout or infectious arthritis appeared. The only way to absolutely rule out infection and definitively diagnose gout, he explained, would be to examine and culture a sample of joint fluid, usually obtained through a needle.

In gout, the inflammation is caused by the formation of monosodium urate crystals in the joint fluid. Sometimes incorrectly referred to as uric acid, monosodium urate (MSU for short) is a breakdown product of cells. It is not very soluble, and when large amounts of it are present in the body fluids, it can crystallize. The body tries to get rid of the MSU crystals by mobilizing specialized cells to swallow them up and carry them off. This leads to inflammation. The crystals have a characteristic needlelike appearance. They polarize light—that is, they are birefringent—and they can be readily identified using a polarizing microscope that employs special filters to determine the direction of polarization of the crystals. The presence of such crystals in the joint fluid is diagnostic of gout.

Elmer was apprehensive, but the doctor reassured him that the pain from aspirating the joint with a needle would be minimal compared to what he was already experiencing. Elmer reluctantly acquiesced to the procedure.

Though further testing would be necessary to confirm the diagnosis, Elmer's doctor indeed detected MSU crystals in his joint fluid, clearly indicating gout. He added that coexisting infection would not be absolutely ruled out until the culture results were reported a day or two later, but he wanted to start gout treatment right away.

How are joint aspirations performed?

First, the doctor will administer a local anesthetic, similar to that used by dentists, into the skin and deeper tissues over the inflamed joint. This will make the procedure less uncomfortable, although the anesthetic may initially produce a short-lived burning sensation. Then he will extract joint fluid through a larger, empty syringe with a bigger needle. Most patients are relieved to find that joint aspiration is less painful than they expected it to be.

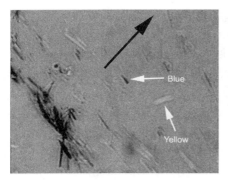

Figure 4-2: Urate crystals photographed through a polarizing microscope with a first-order red filter. The crystals appear yellow (light colored) when they are oriented parallel to the axis of slow vibration (black arrow), and blue (dark) when they are perpendicular to it. This is called negative birefringence, and it is characteristic of urate crystals. Positive birefringence (blue when parallel, yellow when perpendicular to the axis) is characteristic of calcium pyrophosphate dihydrate (CPPD) crystals, found in a condition dubbed pseudogout.

Some of the yellowish fluid will be put into a sterile container for culture and some into a tube for analysis in the lab. Finally, the doctor will examine a drop of fluid from the syringe through a special microscope under polarized light in order to detect the presence of those needlelike MSU crystals.

All about Gout

Of all the ills known to afflict humankind, very few have accumulated a social lore as rich as that associated with gout. Perhaps the only other disease that comes close in this regard is tuberculosis, with its spas in the mountains, where such people as Hans Castorp went for the cure in Thomas Mann's *The Magic Mountain*.

Gout was not only well known throughout recorded history, having been described by Hippocrates in the 5th century B.C., but at times people considered it to be almost a badge of success. In the 15th century, Piero de' Medici, who led the Florentine state until his death, was known as Piero il Gottoso, or Piero the Gouty. Piero's father, Cosimo, and son Lorenzo (the family's most famous scion, dubbed the Magnificent) also were afflicted. Interestingly, more recent investigations have cast some doubt on the correctness of the diagnosis of gout in the de' Medici family, favoring instead ankylosing spondylitis (see chapter 5), an unknown condition at that time.

Cartoons from the 18th and 19th centuries depict the typical afflicted individual as a well-fed, wealthy man surrounded by his minions and retainers, the aggrieved foot generously wrapped in soft cloths soaked with soothing poultices and supported on a cushion, while Rubenesque female attendants lumber about, responding to his every need. In some old prints and cartoons, the devil himself is depicted sticking the painful extremity with a pitchfork.

What causes gout?

As mentioned previously, gout is caused by the build-up of monosodium urate crystals in the joint fluid. Sometimes incorrectly referred to as uric acid, monosodium urate (MSU) is a breakdown product of cell nuclei. It is not very soluble, and when large amounts of it are present in the body fluids, it can crystallize. MSU crystals are highly inflammatory, and the body tries to get rid of them by mobilizing specialized cells to swallow them up and carry them off. This leads to inflammation.

In Elmer's case, the attack was almost certainly provoked by the ingestion of large quantities of alcohol (and probably meat as well), which temporarily increased his MSU level and caused the poorly soluble substance to crystallize. In fact, this sequence of events, observed over the centuries, is likely responsible for the popular association of gout with drinking and gluttony. But plenty of people do the same things that Elmer did without having attacks of gout, so there has to be more to it than that. The underlying process—overproduction of urate—must persist for a long time before there is a sufficient accumulation of crystals to cause an attack.

In other cases, gout attacks may be induced by exposure to lead. The people at greatest risk are those involved in the production and consumption of illegal whiskey, or moonshine, because the home-made stills usually contain lead, which leaches its way into the brew. In these cases it may be a little difficult to tell what is due to lead toxicity and what is due to alcohol, but the lead apparently plays a role, although it is not entirely clear what that role is. Nonetheless, the association is clearly enough recognized that gout associated with lead toxicity has its own special name: saturnine gout.

Sometimes gout attacks occur in people with cancer as they initiate chemotherapy. The chemotherapeutic drugs cause cancer-cell death on a massive scale, and the dead cell nuclei are broken down by normal pathways, resulting in, among other things, high concentrations of the waste product urate. A drug called allopurinol is sometimes used to prevent this problem, but since this agent interacts with certain chemotherapeutic agents, caution is advisable.

Finally, there is evidence that physical trauma can provoke an attack in a joint with extensive urate deposits, possibly by dislodging some crystals into the joint fluid. Some doctors believe that the big toe is a target for gout because of its constant exposure to minor trauma. Proof of this mechanism is limited, but it makes a certain amount of sense.

What tests do I need?

Elmer's doctor explained that four tests are typically performed to diagnose gout:

- Joint-fluid analysis and culture confirm the diagnosis of gout and rule out infection. The specimens are sent to the laboratory for determination of the number and type of inflammatory cells and for culture. Ordinarily, the lab techs look for crystals, but in Elmer's case this was redundant, since the doctor had already found them.

- The blood uric acid (urate) level would probably—but not necessarily—be elevated above normal. The doctor noted that blood urate levels are often lower during acute attacks than at other times in people with gout. In a gout attack, it is the level of urate in the joint, not in the blood, that matters. Urate levels provide targets for treatment after the acute attack settles down. In most laboratories, the normal range goes up to 7 milligrams per deciliter (mg/dL) of blood, but the target for adequate treatment is lower.

- Many doctors have the patient collect a 24-four-hour urine specimen for measuring its urate content. Urate is poorly soluble, especially in an acidic environment like urine, and people who excrete large amounts of it are prone to develop stones in the urinary tract. Since some of the older methods for lowering uric acid in the blood do so by increasing its excretion rate, the 24-hour urinary excretion rate may be useful data in selecting a long-term treatment protocol.

- An X-ray of Elmer's foot was useful because he could not be sure whether or not one of its small bones had been fractured. But given that this was a first attack that had begun less than 24 hours earlier, the erosions typical of long-standing gout were not likely to be present. In gout, X-rays are more useful if there have been repeated attacks or even chronic arthritis. In a bacterially infected (septic) joint, X-ray changes develop over a period of a few days and therefore would not have been expected in Elmer's case at that time.

Many people with gout have other associated conditions, the most frequent being type 2 diabetes and high blood levels of fatty substances called lipids. Although the time for this evaluation is not necessarily during an acute attack, it should be included in a gout sufferer's health maintenance program.

Is gout genetic?

The genetics of common gout are obscure. Elmer was surprised to learn that he had gout, but he was familiar with the disease because his father also had it. According to the National Institute of Arthritis and Musculoskeletal and Skin Diseases (NIAMS), about 18 percent of those with gout can identify other family members with the condition, suggesting the possibility of a hereditary component.

But many other factors affect the likelihood that a given person will develop gout, including:

- Dietary and drinking habits
- Gender (gout is more likely to occur in men)
- Obesity
- Medications such as diuretics, salicylates, niacin, cyclosporine, and levodopa

Does gout predispose me to other diseases?

Conditions associated with an increased incidence of gout include illnesses in which there is rapid cell turnover, such as cancer, especially at the onset of chemotherapy; psoriasis, a common inflammatory skin disorder; sarcoidosis, a tuberculosis-like disease of unknown cause; pseudogout, an arthritic condition caused by precipitation of calcium pyrophosphate crystals in joints; obesity; type 2 diabetes; hypertension; lead poisoning; kidney failure; organ transplantation; and high cholesterol. In some cases the mechanisms are fairly well understood, while in others they remain obscure.

Although allopurinol can prevent attacks of gout, it has no effect on most of these conditions associated with gout, which must be treated separately from gout.

Can gout attacks be prevented?

Since attacks of gout occur when MSU crystals form in the joints, lowering the urate concentration in the blood should reduce the likelihood of a gout attack. There are two main methods for accomplishing this: (1) increasing the rate at which urate is cleared from the bloodstream via the kidneys, and (2) decreasing the rate at which urate is produced.

Increasing urate clearance was the original medical strategy for preventing attacks. One method—not very effective—was making the urine less acidic in order to slightly speed urate's clearance from the circulation. Over the years, physicians developed several methods for doing this, usually involving the ingestion of large amounts of vile-tasting alkalinizing solutions with multisyllabic names. A better method came with the recognition that probenecid, a drug that was originally developed to decrease the rate at which penicillin was cleared from the body, enhanced the clearance rate of urate from the blood. This was the first truly effective method for preventing attacks of gout. Probenecid worked better when the urine was less acidic, so combining these two methods worked better than either one alone.

The more recent, and clearly more effective, strategy is to decrease the rate at which urate enters the bloodstream. An early approach to this was to alter the diet so that there would be less precursor material (purines) for the formation of urate. Although low-purine diets may not be as distasteful as alkalinizing solutions, they are certainly not gourmet delights (see boxed list of foods high in purine content). Luckily, the reduction of urate synthesis is more effectively accomplished by the drug allopurinol, introduced in 1964. This drug blocks one of the enzymes—xanthine oxidase—important in urate production.

An alternative to allopurinol, febuxostat, was introduced in Europe in 2008, making it the first new gout treatment in 40 years. Like allopurinol, it also works by suppressing the action of xanthine oxidase. Febuxostat has not, as of this writing, been approved in the United States.

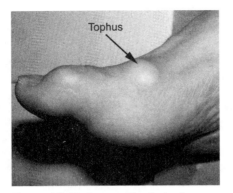

Figure 4-3: Tophus on the foot of a man with long-standing gout.

When MSU-crystal deposits form in the skin, they are called tophi, and the gout is referred to as tophaceous. But similar deposits build up in the joint membranes, and by the time an acute attack occurs, they will have been forming for months to years. Paradoxically, people taking allopurinol may still suffer attacks at first. As the medication begins to dissolve the crystal deposits, MSU particles may break away from the tissues to which they have become anchored, float free in the joint fluid, and cause inflammation. For that reason, during the early months of treatment it is advisable to take a small dose of colchicine, an antigout agent, or an NSAID—but generally not both—to prevent attacks until all the urate deposits are dissolved out of the joints and tissues. This may take 6 to 12 months, after which the anti-inflammatory treatment—colchicine or NSAID—can usually be discontinued. Allopurinol, however, must be taken permanently, or else the attacks of gout will resume.

Can diet help?

The stereotypical image of the gluttonous, fat, middle-aged male with gout suggests that a more spartan, less excessive lifestyle may reduce the likelihood of the disease. Although this image is perhaps a bit overplayed, the so-called metabolic syndrome, or syndrome X, encompasses high blood lipids, hypertension, abdominal obesity, and type 2 diabetes. Gout often occurs in this setting.

As mentioned previously, a low-purine diet can help reduce the frequency of attacks. Foods high in purines include organ meats, certain seafood, game fowl, meat extracts, and dried legumes. Avoid the following foods, and you'll reduce your chances of suffering attacks.

Foods High in Purine Content

Organ Meats

- Brain
- Liver
- Heart
- Kidneys
- Sweetbreads (pancreas, thymus)

Game Fowl

- Goose
- Partridge

Meat Extracts

- Gravy
- Broth
- Bouillon
- Consomme

Seafood

- Mackerel
- Herring
- Shrimp
- Mussels
- Scallops
- Anchovies
- Sardines
- Roe

Dried Legumes

- Dried beans
- Dried peas

Beneficial foods include those that decrease the acidity of the urine, such as fruit juices, especially cherry juice; rice; many vegetables; and dairy products.

Should I exercise if I have gout?

Exercise would be impossible during an acute gout attack. At other times, though, you should be able to exercise without difficulty.

How common is gout?

Gout affects about 6.1 million Americans.

Treating Gout

Depending on the situation, there are several choices for initial treatment of an acute gout attack. The most rapid and complete resolution of an acute attack can usually be accomplished by using two agents.

The first is ACTH (adrenocorticotropic hormone), injected into muscle tissue, which rapidly and completely resolves the acute arthritis of gout. However, it provides but a temporary solution, lasting about a day. ACTH is a hormone produced by the pituitary gland, a small gland at the base of the brain. Its primary effect is to stimulate the adrenal glands to produce cortisone. You may be wondering why, if that's the case, a gout patient wouldn't simply be given prednisone, a synthetic cortisone drug. Many physicians who treat gout believe that ACTH has other beneficial effects, not well understood, that make it work better than oral cortisone or prednisone. In many cases, the injection has to be repeated a day later, but generally not beyond that.

The second medication is indomethacin or another fast-acting nonsteroidal anti-inflammatory drug such as ibuprofen, diclofenac, and others. These have a less potent but longer-lasting suppressive effect on acute inflammation. This medication should be taken at the same time as the first dose of ACTH and continued for ten days to two weeks. Needless to say, you should take all drugs at their recommended dosages

The classic treatment is colchicine alone, without ACTH or NSAIDs. Colchicine is a derivative of a naturally occurring chemical found in the autumn crocus. Colchicine tablets, which can be taken at the rate of one per hour until diarrhea inevitably occurs, often cool down an acute attack of gout. In many cases, however, this just replaces the problem of gout with the problem of diarrhea, and the use of oral colchicine for acute attacks has, for the most part, joined the ranks of historical treatments that have been replaced by better approaches. Colchicine can also be administered intravenously—its current main use in this form is to treat patients with acute gout who can't take oral medications. This might be the case, for example, during the period immediately after an operation requiring general anesthesia, a common time for a first gout attack in those who are prone to the disorder.

Can gout be cured?

There is no known cure for gout, but most cases can be controlled completely using prophylactic, or preventive, medication.

What factors are considered when choosing a treatment plan?

Since medications are used to treat both acute attacks and to prevent new attacks, it is important to make sure that you can tolerate the drugs. You should not be allergic to NSAIDs or have impaired kidney function or other contraindications to the use of these drugs. You should not be taking azathioprine, which interferes with allopurinol, or drugs that alter the activity of NSAIDs.

What are the side effects of these treatments?

ACTH, cortisone, and prednisone all suppress the body's ability to fend off infection. If these drugs are administered to someone with an existing, undiagnosed infection, the result can be disastrous, with infection spreading rapidly and destructively. Other acute side effects include fluid retention, flushing, and steroid psychosis—an agitated or euphoric state induced by taking cortisonelike drugs. For reasons nobody understands, the exact symptoms vary in different people. These drugs can also acutely disrupt control of diabetes.

NSAID side effects include gastric irritation, headache, ringing in the ears (tinnitus), dizziness, asthma, kidney failure, and high blood pressure. Most of these occur more frequently in older people. In addition, these drugs interact with certain other medications, such as the blood thinner warfarin, causing them to behave unexpectedly at their usual doses.

Finally, colchicine causes diarrhea, vomiting, and sometimes suppression of blood cell production.

Elmer's Treatment

Medication

After ascertaining that Elmer had no history of peptic ulcer disease, asthma, or kidney disease, and that he was not taking medications for anything else, the doctor recommended ACTH, 80 units injected into the muscle, and 50 milligrams of indomethacin three times daily with meals. He scheduled Elmer for a return visit the next day to evaluate the response and to give another ACTH injection if necessary. The attack resolved in a few hours, and Elmer felt normal again. Since an acute attack of gout normally lasts only a few days whether it is treated or not, once it has cleared up, attention should turn to how to prevent another attack.

Elmer's Response to Treatment

Within a few hours of receiving ACTH and starting indomethacin, Elmer felt "ninety-five percent better," and by the next day, after receiving the second dose of ACTH, he was completely recovered.

The doctor told him that he still had gout, but that taking allopurinol could probably prevent future attacks. Specifically, he recommended that Elmer follow this regimen:

- Start allopurinol at 100 milligrams daily for seven days; then increase the dose to 200 milligrams daily for another seven days; then increase the dose to 300 milligrams daily and continue that dose indefinitely.
- Start colchicine at 0.6 milligrams twice daily and continue for six months.

What to Expect

Will I be disabled?

Elmer's diagnosis was made soon after the onset of the first attack. In that setting, there is usually little if any joint destruction, and crippling does not occur. However, sometimes gout is not diagnosed or properly treated early, and that's when a chronic destructive form can develop. This condition resembles chronic active rheumatoid arthritis in many people. In its intermediate and late stages, chronic gouty arthritis can be diagnosed by examining the joint fluid under polarized light microscopy, and treatment, as already described, can halt the progression of the disease but some damage may remain. This damage may lead to impaired function of the involved joints. It would be quite rare, however, for gouty arthritis to lead to the need for reconstructive surgery on affected joints.

Elmer's Outcome

It would be nice to be able to say that Elmer could expect to live happily ever after. That would probably be a fair prognosis with respect to his gout, but gout seldom exists in a vacuum. Elmer's turbocharged

Disease at a Glance: Gout

Who Gets It?

- Men more than women
- Associated with type A personality
- Weak heredity component
- 2.1 million Americans affected in a given year; over 6 million have had at least one attack

Joint Involvement

- Typically affects one joint but sometimes strikes more than one
- Most characteristic: big toe
- Typical length of acute attacks: three to five days

Other Features and Complications

- Tophi
- Kidney stones
- If not treated, leads to chronic arthritis of multiple joints
- May be associated with sarcoidosis, psoriasis, metabolic syndrome

Lab Results

- Elevated blood uric acid
- Needlelike monosodium urate crystals in joint fluid
- Often increased uric acid excretion in urine

Treatment

- Acute attack
  - Colchicine or NSAID
  - ACTH or systemic corticosteroid (such as prednisone)
- Preventive maintenance
  - Allopurinol or other urate-lowering medication
  - Avoiding dietary indiscretions
  - Adequate fluid intake
  - Education

lifestyle carried with it a variety of hazards going far beyond the health of his joints.

The doctor noted that Elmer probably either had or was at risk for the metabolic syndrome. This all-too-common condition is the combination of central (abdominal) obesity, high blood pressure, insulin resistance (including type 2 diabetes), and abnormal blood lipids. Individuals with metabolic syndrome often have gout along with it. More ominously, metabolic syndrome is also associated with hardening of the arteries (atherosclerosis), heart attacks, and strokes. Although it certainly got Elmer's attention, gout would probably be the least of his problems in the long run.

Chapter 5

Ankylosing Spondylitis and Reactive Arthritis

Onset: Oh, My Aching Back!

Clyde awoke to the rustling murmur of a soft wind outside his open window, gently disturbing the curtains. It was still dark, but he was having trouble sleeping; as had been the case for the last couple of months, his back was bothering him. He tried shifting to a new position but couldn't get comfortable. Not only was his back sore, but it was stiff as well. He opened his burning eyes and looked at his clock: 3:00 A.M. In about 30 minutes, the alarm would go off, and he would have to get up anyway to study for a histology examination that he was scheduled to take a few hours later. Might as well just get up and be done with it.

At age 22, Clyde was in his second year of medical school, and he couldn't get over how lucky he was. He was the fifth of 12 children. They had all grown up on the family farm in Clarke County, Iowa. Although they always had enough to eat and inexpensive but serviceable

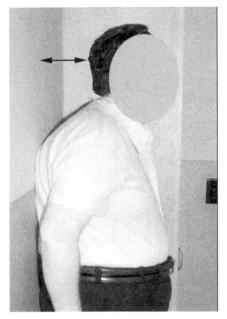

Figure 5-1: Middle-aged man with moderately advanced ankylosing spondylitis. When he stands with his heels against the wall, he can't touch his head to the wall. Head-to-wall distance, finger-to-floor distance, and chest expansion are classical measurements for following the progress of the disease.

clothes to wear, money was perennially tight; and with Dad disabled by arthritis of his back, the kids had to pitch in to get the work done, bring in the crops, and tend to the livestock. When Clyde's older brothers, Wilbur and Clarence, also started complaining of back pain and scaled back their contributions to the effort, Clyde and the younger kids had even more to do. It was hard work, especially at certain times of the year, and the vulnerability of the family fortunes to the bodily infirmities of key players made an indelible impression on young Clyde. He resolved early on to get into a line of work that would make him a little less dependent on his physical strength and robust health.

Hard study and scholarships had gotten him through his undergraduate courses at Iowa State and from there to the University of Iowa medical school, where he was now toiling his way through the hardest academic work he had ever known. He was looking forward to getting to the clinical subject matter, especially back pain. Maybe he would be able to figure out the family curse. Old Doc Utterback called it "the rheumatiz," but Clyde thought somehow there might be more to it than that.

Painfully and slowly, he began the daily ritual of getting himself out of bed. There was nothing unusual about the back stiffness, but the pain in his eyes added a new dimension to his discomfort. Within a minute or two, Clyde was able to stand up, but he was unable to straighten completely for about ten minutes, making his way to the bathroom with a hunched posture that made him think of Quasimodo.

Gradually, as Clyde brushed his teeth, he stretched himself upright. Even deep breathing hurt his back. After a few minutes, when he could position his head so that he could see himself in the mirror, a rheumy, bloodshot pair of eyes stared back at him. "God, I look like a case from 'The Crypt of Terror,'" Clyde muttered grimly. "I wonder what that's all about." In the end, it was the new problem with his painful, red eyes that scared him. He could live with the back pain, but he didn't relish the thought of trying to practice medicine blind. He went to the student infirmary as soon as he could get himself moving and asked to see the doctor on call.

Clyde's Assessment

The doctor running the student health clinic was not much older than Clyde, but he was a nice guy and seemed to know what he was doing. He asked Clyde about his symptoms and appeared interested not only in his eyes but also in his back. It hadn't occurred to Clyde that the two problems might be related. The doctor also seemed interested in the fact that Clyde's father and two of his brothers had similar back problems. He asked Clyde about some symptoms that he *hadn't* had: rash, mouth ulcers, and, to Clyde's further surprise, discharge from the penis. Then he performed a brief examination, focusing on Clyde's eyes and back.

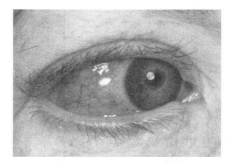

"Well, Clyde, I'm not entirely sure," the young doctor finally said, "but I think you have ankylosing spondylitis, and it appears to be complicated by the presence of an inflammatory condition in your eyes called iritis."

Figure 5-2: Iritis in a patient with ankylosing spondylitis. Note the prominently dilated blood vessels over the white portion of the eye. This condition, which is also seen in reactive arthritis, is potentially highly damaging to the eye and requires aggressive treatment to avoid visual impairment.

Ankylosing spondylitis is caused by inflammation in the joints of the spine. It may lead to fusion—ankylosis—of the spinal vertebrae. It's a fairly common form of arthritis, and the susceptibility to it is inherited in a predictable pattern.

Iritis, which refers to inflammation in the pigmented layer of the eyes, occasionally occurs in association with ankylosing spondylitis. It's a serious condition that needs to be diagnosed and treated without delay in order to relieve pain and protect the vision. Clyde's doctor scheduled him for some blood tests and X-rays, then sent him immediately to see the clinic's ophthalmologist to determine the exact nature of what was going on in his eyes.

After a thorough examination, the ophthalmologist agreed with the young doctor's diagnosis of iritis. Luckily, there didn't appear to be any permanent damage, so she gave Clyde a prescription for some cortisone eyedrops and instructed him to return in a few days. "If at any time you think your eyes are getting worse, especially if you feel you are losing vision," she said, "call me right away."

A couple of days later, his eyes much improved and feeling good about having passed his histology exam, Clyde went back to the student health clinic to go over the lab and X-ray results with the young doctor. With the doctor was an older man, whom the young doctor introduced, saying, "He is my rheumatology professor, and I have asked him to join us today to give us some advice on what to do."

The rheumatologist shook hands with Clyde. He reported that the tests and X-rays confirmed the diagnosis of ankylosing spondylitis. Although Clyde had lost some motion in the lower back, nothing on the films indicated that the disease had progressed to the point where he couldn't regain a lot of this motion with appropriate treatment.

Using a model, he demonstrated to Clyde the parts of the pelvis. He showed him how, on the X-rays, the sacroiliac joints of his pelvis were affected. There appeared to be increased bone density along the margins of these joints and some narrowing and irregularity of the joint space. The rheumatologist explained that the pelvis consists of three pairs of bones: the ilia (wings of the pelvis), ischia (the bones you sit on), and the pubis (the small bones in the front of the pelvic girdle). The ilia are connected to the sacrum (the lowest vertebrae of the spinal column) through the sacroiliac joints, and the pubic bones connect through a similar joint (pubic symphysis) in the front of the pelvic girdle. The sacroiliac joints and the pubic symphysis are fibrous joints with little or no motion under normal circumstances, as opposed to synovial joints like the knees and hips, which move freely. The sacroiliac joints tend to become inflamed in ankylosing spondylitis and generally show the earliest changes that are visible on X-ray in this condition.

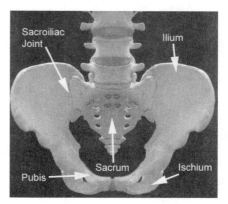

Figure 5-3: Front view of the pelvis of an anatomical model of the human skeleton. In ankylosing spondylitis, the earliest joints to be affected are the sacroiliac joints, which connect the pelvis to the spine.

The rheumatologist noted that although the diagnosis was pretty clear from the symptoms and the sacroiliac joint abnormalities, more X-ray abnormalities would probably be forthcoming, including calcification of the long ligaments at the front and rear of the spine, possibly leading to fusion and the dramatic appearance of the "bamboo spine," so called because it appears like a bamboo branch or stem, that characterizes advanced ankylosing spondylitis.

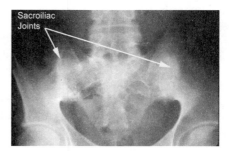

Figure 5-4: X-ray of the pelvis in a patient with moderately advanced ankylosing spondylitis. The bone immediately surrounding the sacroiliac joints is sclerotic—that is, densely overgrown and white in appearance on the X-ray, because of stimulation by the presence of inflammation in the joints. The end result of this activity is generally fusion of the sacroiliac joints.

One of the most important aspects of treating ankylosing spondylitis is to avoid having

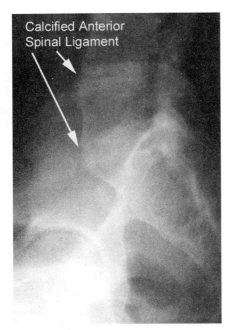

Calcified Anterior
Spinal Ligament

Figure 5-5: X-ray of a side (lateral) view of the lower (lumbosacral) spine in a patient with ankylosing spondylitis, showing some characteristics of the typical bamboo spine. Note the calcium in the front spinal ligament, most easily seen in front of the joints between the vertebrae.

the spine fuse in a forward-flexed position. If that should happen, it may become impossible for the person to look up high enough to see the horizon.

The rheumatologist also took note of the fact that one of Clyde's blood tests, the HLA-B27 test, was positive.

All about Ankylosing Spondylitis

What are the symptoms of ankylosing spondylitis?

The hallmark of ankylosing spondylitis (AS) is low back pain and stiffness, which tends to be worse at rest. It typically wakes you up in the early morning hours and gets a little better if you walk around. The disorder often restricts forward flexion of the spine, making it difficult to bend and touch your toes. It may also restrict neck motion, so that the head tends to remain in a looking-down position. Ankylosing spondylitis typically afflicts young men, although it can affect women, usually less severely. It can affect your peripheral joints, such as the hips and knees, but it is less likely to involve the hands and wrists.

What tests do I need?

A positive HLA-B27 test does not have a high specificity for the diagnosis, since only 1 percent of such people have ankylosing spondylitis severe enough to treat. But since almost all Caucasians with ankylosing spondylitis have a positive HLA-B27 test, a negative result would be strong evidence against the diagnosis.

HLA-B27 blood tests are almost always positive in Caucasians with ankylosing spondylitis, although a positive test does not always indicate that you have the disease. HLA-B27 (the HLA stands for human leukocyte antigen) is like a blood type, except that the antigen is found on the surface of white blood cells rather than on red cells. About 5 to 8 percent of Caucasians are positive for HLA-B27; it is much rarer in African-Americans and almost does not occur at all in pure African blacks. Most ethnic Asian populations have HLA-B27 in about the same proportions as whites: 5 to 10 percent in the general population and 95 percent in patients with ankylosing spondylitis. Recent research has focused on the 25 or so subtypes of HLA-B27, which are distributed differently in various ethnic groups. The practical significance of this finding remains to be determined.

In Clyde's case, the clinical evidence in favor of the diagnosis was so strong that the HLAB27 result had minor confirmatory value in making the diagnosis. If the test result had been negative, however, the doctor might have gone back to the drawing board to look for other causes of his patient's symptoms.

Does ankylosing spondylitis affect only the spine?

Although ankylosing spondylitis always affects the spine, including the lumbar (lower back region), thoracic (chest region), and cervical (neck region) spine, in some people it affects other joints as well, especially the peripheral joints of the lower extremities. Hip involvement is fairly common and may be severe, and almost any joint may occasionally become inflamed in this disease. Unlike with rheumatoid arthritis, however, such joint activity is often asymmetrical. While rheumatoid arthritis tends to affect both hips symmetrically, ankylosing spondylitis might affect just one, or it might affect both with greatly differing severity. Nevertheless, like rheumatoid arthritis, this peripheral joint form of ankylosing spondylitis can be very destructive, frequently leading to surgery.

Does ankylosing spondylitis affect parts of the body other than joints?

Ankylosing spondylitis is a systemic disease that may involve various organ systems, though arthritis is generally the most prominent component. As we see with Clyde's case, it can also affect the eyes. It can cause painful ulcerations in the mouth and nose. It may also be accompanied by a heart murmur due to a leaky aortic valve (aortic insufficiency), or by an aneurysm—a weakening of the wall—of the great artery known as the aorta. These aneurysms can rupture with disastrous results. Fortunately, this doesn't occur very often.

Does ankylosing spondylitis predispose me to other diseases?

HLA-B27 is interesting. Since the association with ankylosing spondylitis became apparent in the mid-1970s, several diseases that had not been previously linked on clinical grounds were found to have a high frequency of HLA-B27 positivity. Prior to that, ankylosing spondylitis was considered to be a form of rheumatoid arthritis and was often called rheumatoid spondylitis. Ankylosing spondylitis and related entities are now commonly referred to as the seronegative spondyloarthropathies.

The term seronegative means that, as a group, patients with these conditions do not have positive rheumatoid factor tests (see chapter 2). Besides ankylosing spondylitis, the seronegative spondyloarthropathies include:

- Reactive arthritis, which is sometimes called Reiter's syndrome in the United States and Germany, and Fiessinger-Leroy syndrome in France;
- Psoriatic arthritis with spondylitis;
- Enteropathic arthritis with spondylitis; and
- Some cases of seronegative rheumatoid arthritis, which have also been called incomplete Reiter's syndrome.

What is Reiter's syndrome?

Classical Reiter's syndrome refers to the combination of (1) arthritis; (2) inflammation of the urethra not caused by gonorrhea, or nongonococcal urethritis; and (3) inflammation of certain eye structures, such as iritis or uveitis. If any of the three components is absent, the term incomplete Reiter's syndrome would be used. The syndrome sometimes occurs in the setting of a urinary tract infection; a sexually transmitted infection, especially chlamydia; or a diarrheal gastrointestinal infection, as with salmonella or shigella. It may be acute or chronic, and people with HLA-B27 are markedly more susceptible to the chronic form of it than those who lack this genetic marker.

The name Reiter's syndrome is actually in the process of being phased out in favor of the much more descriptive *reactive arthritis*. Reiter was a German physician who wrote an early description of the condition. In fact, Reiter wasn't the first to describe reactive arthritis or the triad of symptoms that bears his name. The new designation recognizes this while tacitly acknowledging recently publicized evidence about Reiter's activities in Germany as an official of the Third Reich.

Can ankylosing spondylitis and reactive arthritis be prevented?

Ankylosing spondylitis and reactive arthritis are genetically based disorders and probably can't be prevented. Reactive arthritis may require an infection, usually genitourinary or gastrointestinal, as a trigger for an initial attack.

Can diet help?

There is no known benefit to any dietary intervention in the seronegative spondyloarthropathies.

Should I exercise if I have ankylosing spondylitis?

Exercise in the form of a formal physical therapy program is extremely important in managing ankylosing spondylitis; in fact, it's the core of treatment. Staying active preserves flexibility of the spine. This tends to be a losing battle over time unless the disease goes into a spontaneous remission or is aggressively treated with anti-inflammatory medication. But without an exercise program, you'll lose more mobility more quickly. The second purpose of physical therapy is to ensure that, in the event that you lose mobility, the spine does not fuse in an extreme forward-flexed or twisted position, which, as you can imagine, becomes enormously disabling.

How common are ankylosing spondylitis and reactive arthritis?

The prevalence of these conditions is not known with certainty, partially because many people apparently have mild, untreated forms. Estimates range up to about 2 million Americans. Ankylosing spondylitis manifests in all degrees of severity, from very mild and almost without symptoms to extremely severe and disabling. About 20 percent of people with HLA-B27 have some evidence of ankylosing spondylitis, but only about 1 percent of people with HLA-B27 develop ankylosing spondylitis symptoms severe enough to require treatment.

Treating Ankylosing Spondylitis and Reactive Arthritis

Treatment of ankylosing spondylitis has three components:

- Exercise and physical therapy to maintain mobility
- Medications to control inflammation and pain
- Surgery to correct damaged joints

If other organ systems, such as the eyes or the blood vessels, are involved, specific treatments for these manifestations need to be considered as well.

Treatment of reactive arthritis is the same as treatment of the peripheral joint manifestations of ankylosing spondylitis.

Can ankylosing spondylitis and reactive arthritis be cured?

There is no cure for ankylosing spondylitis, and it has to be treated as a chronic disease. The same is true of reactive arthritis. Fortunately, with new medications, the outlook is a little brighter for people with the more severe forms of these diseases.

What factors are considered when choosing a treatment plan?

Treatment must be tailored to the parts of the body affected and the level of disease activity. Highly active disease, as indicated by severity and acuteness of symptoms, findings on examination, and certain laboratory abnormalities, requires aggressive medical treatment along the same lines as rheumatoid arthritis (see chapter 2). In reactive arthritis, if there is urinary or gastrointestinal infection, antibiotics may be warranted if the organism can be identified.

Clyde's Treatment

Clyde's rheumatologist referred him to a physical medicine and rehabilitation specialist, Dr. Nelson, who would design an appropriate exercise program and instruct him on what he needed to do to remain limber. The new doctor also advised Clyde to start taking 500 milligrams of the NSAID naproxen twice daily with food.

How are ankyklosing spondylitis and reactive arthritis treated

We typically treat patients with the spondyloarthropathies using medications and physical therapy. Surgery is necessary for a minority of patients.

Medications As noted above, the basis of a good treatment program is an NSAID, such as naproxen, in full dosage, as in Clyde's case. Any of the NSAIDs may be used but naproxen combines a relatively good safety profile with reasonable convenience (twice-a-day dosing).

The most common side effects of naproxen are upset stomach, ringing of the ears (tinnitus), kidney impairment, fluid retention, and hypertension. It may also cause easy bruising. Prolonged use may lead to peptic ulcer formation and gastrointestinal bleeding, diarrhea, and, in some people, impaired liver function. No medicine is completely safe, but as anti-inflammatory drugs go, naproxen isn't too bad. It's important, however, that your doctor monitors your progress on the drug to make sure it doesn't adversely affect you.

The antimetabolic drug methotrexate, the standard of treatment for rheumatoid arthritis, is not as effective for ankylosing spondylitis, but it has proved beneficial for some patients. It would generally be added as second-line therapy if the response to the NSAID is unsatisfactory. It, too, requires monitoring (see chapter 2).

Tumor necrosis factor–alpha (TNF-alpha) inhibitors may be the long-awaited breakthrough that allows us to treat most cases of ankylosing spondylitis effectively. The early results with these drugs (etanercept, infliximab, and adalimumab) are very encouraging, and they do not seem to have insurmountable short-term toxicity. Only time will tell how well people tolerate them over the long haul.

The same strategy applies to treating reactive arthritis with medications. If an infection of the urinary tract or gastrointestinal tract can be identified, your physician will treat you with an appropriate antibiotic. This may improve the arthritis as well as clearing up local symptoms (urethral discharge or diarrhea). Otherwise, reactive arthritis requires much the same approach as rheumatoid arthritis.

Physical therapy Nowhere is physical therapy more important than in the treatment of ankylosing spondylitis. The basic program consists of active exercises to maintain range of motion in the spine and to stretch and strengthen muscles. The use of passive modalities such as heat, diathermy, and the like plays a role only in preparing for the active exercise modalities. Depending on the areas of greatest disease activity, as determined by physical examination and X-rays, the professional (physiatrist or physical therapist) will design a specific program tailored to the patient's needs.

Surgery Many people with ankylosing spondylitis also develop peripheral joint inflammation, especially in the hips, knees, and ankles, and this is typically treated like rheumatoid arthritis. Most orthopedic surgical procedures performed for patients with ankylosing spondylitis are aimed at peripheral joint disease. Hip and knee replacement surgery and ankle fusions are common procedures performed on patients with ankylosing spondylitis. Clyde might eventually become a candidate for this kind of reconstructive surgery.

Surgery on the spine is fraught with hazard and in this disease is best avoided if possible. Furthermore, any surgery requiring general anesthesia is difficult when the neck is locked into a bent-forward position. This can make it almost impossible to insert a breathing tube, which must be in place while the patient is anesthetized.

Clyde's Response to Treatment

As initial treatment, Clyde started taking naproxen, 500 milligrams twice daily with food. After about ten days, he noticed that the stiffness he experienced in the mornings was somewhat reduced in severity and duration. He also had less soreness in his back, though he certainly was not symptom-free.

Dr. Nelson, the physiatrist, was a kindly, elderly man with an interest in medical history, and Clyde enjoyed talking to him. The physiatrist explained that the so-called passive modalities of physical therapy (deep heat, diathermy, ultrasound) might provide some minimal and very temporary relief, enabling Clyde to do the active exercises more effectively. The main benefits, however, would come from active exercise, particularly stretching.

Dr. Nelson wrote out a physical therapy prescription and literally put Clyde into the hands of a blonde woman named Inga. Clyde figured that he had better cooperate, since Inga looked as if she could throttle him if she had to. After applying moist heat to his back for a few minutes, Inga showed Clyde how to do the stretching and strengthening back exercises and watched him go through a few repetitions. He felt better immediately, and for the first time, he began to feel somewhat optimistic about how his treatment was going. Inga smiled and patted him on the head. "You feel better, no?" Clyde nodded, to which she responded, "Good. Go home now and do it."

What happens if treatment stops working?

If the first line of medication doesn't work, there are other medications to try and even surgeries to perform. Eventually, as we learn more about the long-term effects of new drugs, the treatment protocols may change. Drugs such as the TNF-alpha inhibitors may become first-line treatments, not only for ankylosing spondylitis but for many other forms of arthritis as well.

For now, however, if we can get satisfactory control of the disease with drugs that are more familiar, that is preferable. Along with physical therapy, this is a common, safe, and often effective way to begin a treatment plan.

Complications and first follow-up visit

For the next six weeks, Clyde did his exercises and took his medicine faithfully. Although his back felt better, he was beginning to have a gurgling sensation in his stomach and persistent abdominal pain, sometimes burning, other times cramping. His stools first became soft, then watery at times, and finally black and tarry in appearance and consistency. Bowel movements were explosive, accompanied by voluminous gaseous emanations, and required extensive bathroom cleanup. He began to suspect that all might not be well with his medication, so he returned to the student health clinic.

The internist asked about Clyde's symptoms and suggested that he perform a rectal examination in order to test the stool for blood. The stool sample tested positive for blood. The fact that the stool was black and tarry suggested that the blood was coming from the upper GI tract—that is, the stomach or upper small intestine; blood from the lower tract, or large intestine, would be red. Like all nonselective nonsteroidal anti-inflammatory drugs, naproxen can cause gastritis or ulcers in the stomach and upper small intestine. It can also cause diarrhea.

The doctor outlined the following plan for Clyde:

- First, stop the naproxen.

- Second, schedule an endoscopic examination of the esophagus, stomach, and duodenum (upper small intestine) to check for an ulcer or significant inflammation in that part of the gastrointestinal tract.

- Third, start a new medication called omeprazole to inhibit acid secretion in the stomach; this would promote healing of the problem in the upper tract.

- Fourth, he prescribed loperamide, a medication to control the diarrhea. Clyde would not need to take it for very long, because stopping the naproxen would resolve the diarrhea relatively quickly if that were the cause.

Sometimes inflammatory bowel disease occurs in association with ankylosing spondylitis and other seronegative spondyloarthropathies, and it was possible that could be playing a role in Clyde's situation. "We'll see how discontinuing the naproxen affects the diarrhea and proceed accordingly," the doctor said. "If the diarrhea doesn't stop, we'll need to do a colonoscopy."

Flare-up and second follow-up visit

The combination of stopping naproxen and starting omeprazole and loperamide quickly resolved Clyde's gastrointestinal symptoms. The upper endoscopy (often called EGD, short for esophagogastroduodenoscopy) showed only some irritation of the stomach lining, but there was no evidence of an ulcer. The diarrhea cleared almost immediately when the naproxen was stopped, as did the upper abdominal pain. Clyde's physician discontinued the loperamide and omeprazole after a couple of weeks without the abdominal pain and diarrhea recurring. But the ankylosing spondylitis symptoms came back with a vengeance.

About a month later, Clyde was in the rheumatologist's office with low back pain and stiffness almost as bad as when he had first consulted the internist. After performing a brief examination, the rheumatologist confirmed that the spondylitis was more active again. He asked if Clyde was still doing his exercises. He was, but he found that they were harder to do now than when he was on medication for the arthritis.

"Okay," said the rheumatologist, "here's what we are going to do next.

"First, I want you to start another anti-inflammatory drug, one that is a specific inhibitor of the enzyme cyclooxygenase 2, or COX-2, called celecoxib. This medication is designed to go easy on the gastrointestinal tract. I want you to take one tablet twice daily with food.

"Second, I want you to start methotrexate, a chemotherapy drug that works by inhibiting the body's use of the B vitamin folic acid. This drug also inhibits inflammation by slowing the reproduction of inflammatory cells. Take five tablets each Monday. Methotrexate takes several weeks to work, so don't expect dramatic benefits overnight, but the celecoxib works a little faster and should help some within a few days. When you come back for your next checkup in eight weeks, we'll see how you are doing and check your blood for toxicity of these drugs. In the meantime, I want you to continue your exercises."

Partial improvement and third follow-up visit

Over the next few weeks, Clyde's stiffness improved and his pain lessened. He was able to exercise again without much difficulty. He seemed to tolerate the new medications well. He didn't really feel well, but he was functioning and able to go to his classes without great difficulty. His improvement had been so gradual that he hardly noticed it until he recalled how he'd felt before. He estimated that he had improved about 50 percent. He still couldn't touch the floor with his knees straight, but instead of missing it by a foot, which had been the case previously, he could now get his fingertips to within six inches of the floor. If he stood with his back to the wall, heels touching the baseboard, he could touch the back of his head to the wall with some difficulty and very little pain.

Clyde reported this improvement on his next visit to the rheumatologist and asked, "Is it possible to do any better than this? I still feel sort of sick, and I don't have much energy. I always feel like I'm on the brink of disaster, but I keep on rolling along."

Until a couple of years ago, there wasn't much more to do for ankylosing spondylitis than what Clyde was doing. Most people would improve somewhat. But in difficult cases, and especially in situations where people didn't tolerate the medicines well, the outcomes were unsatisfactory. Now, however, for people who have tried the first and even second lines of defense and still aren't doing well, we have some new, powerful biological agents.

These TNF-alpha inhibitors, which we discussed earlier, block the action of an important inflammatory mediator, tumor necrosis factor-alpha. TNF-alpha inhibitors have recently been shown to be very useful in treating ankylosing spondylitis. In many patients, their effectiveness is little short of miraculous. The drawbacks are that they're very expensive, must be given by injection, and have unknown long-term side effects. Short-term side effects are not particularly common, but they include headache, cough, pain at the injection site, and increased susceptibility to infection. And they have recently been found in a few patients to unmask latent, unsuspected tuberculosis.

This is why doctors tend to pursue all other courses of action first. Before prescribing a TNF-alpha inhibitor, your doctor will order you a skin test called a PPD test to make sure that you have no evidence of tuberculosis. Once it's clear that there's no TB lurking in your body, your doctor will start you on etanercept injections. In Clyde's case, the prescription was for 50 milligrams injected weekly.

Clyde's Outcome

Two months later, Clyde had a spring in his step. He hadn't felt this good in years. Furthermore, he had passed his semester finals with commendations. He literally danced into his rheumatologist's office.

"Hey, Doc, look what I can do!"

He bent forward from the waist and touched his knuckles to the floor with no apparent strain.

The doctor commented dryly, "Now you can carry your knuckles close to the ground just like a normal medical student."

For Clyde, the future may be considerably brighter than it is for his brothers Wilbur and Clarence. Both of them have advanced ankylosing spondylitis with bamboo-spine changes on X-ray and major areas of fusion of the spine in a forward-flexed position. Poor Clarence can't even watch TV in a normal sitting position.

Disease at a Glance: Ankylosing Spondylitis

Who Gets It?

- Earlier onset and harsher symptoms in men than in women
- Strong family history

Joint Involvement

- Sacroiliac and intervertebral joints of the spine
- Bamboo spine
- Late involvement of peripheral joints (especially the hip, knee, or ankle)

Other Features and Complications

- Uveitis/iritis (eye inflammation)
- Aortitis and aortic valve disease (similar to syphilitic vascular disease)

Lab Results

- HLA-B27 positive in more than 90 percent of affected Caucasians
- Acute-phase reactants (sedimentation rate and C-reactive protein) elevated
- Negative blood test for rheumatoid factor

Treatment

- General
  - Adequate rest
  - Exercise to maintain spinal flexibility and other appropriate physical therapy
  - Education
- Medications
  - Aspirin or other NSAID
  - Methotrexate and/or other DMARD
  - TNF-alpha inhibitor
- Surgery if appropriate

Disease at a Glance: Reactive Arthritis

Who Gets It?

- Males more frequently than females
- Strong heredity factor
- May follow urinary tract infection or intestinal infection

Joint Involvement

- Tends to affect only a few joints
- May be destructive

Other Features and Complications

- Iritis/uveitis
- Nongonococcal urethritis
- Psoriasis-like skin rash (keratodermia blenorrhagica)
- Mouth sores

Lab Results

- HLA-B27 usually positive in chronic cases
- Negative blood test for rheumatoid factor
- Acute-phase reactants (sedimentation rate and C-reactive protein) often elevated
- Evidence of shigella or salmonella in stool; chlamydia in urine

Treatment

- General
  — Adequate rest
  — Appropriate exercise
  — Education
- Medications for arthritis
  — Aspirin or other NSAID
  — Methotrexate and/or other DMARD
  — TNF-alpha inhibitor, such as etanercept
  — Local joint injections of corticosteroid

(continued)

- Medications for uveitis/iritis
  — Corticosteroid eyedrops
- Medications for urethritis
  — Appropriate antibiotic, based on culture
- Surgery if appropriate

But through careful attention to exercise and medication, Clyde's ankylosing spondylitis does not seem to have produced any permanent anatomical changes in his spine in two years. There are many questions, nevertheless, about how well Clyde will do over the long run. Will the etanercept, along with his other treatments, continue to hold the disease in check? Will he eventually be able to stop some or all of his medications? Will etanercept produce undesirable long-term side effects that we can only guess at now? And what is the future of celecoxib? We don't know. So far, however, things look good. As with all new treatments, vigilance—on the part of both physician and patient—is the key to long-term safety and success.

Chapter 6

Psoriatic Arthritis

Onset: The Heartbreak of Psoriasis May Be a Joint Venture

It was two o'clock on a February morning, and Ralph's trio was just finishing its last set. The air in the bar was heavy with stale cigarette smoke, although only a couple of customers remained. Ralph laid down a few final riffs at the keyboard, scratched his itching scalp, and signaled the group to pack it in. He would be glad to get home that night. The gig had been a bummer. The small "crowd" was dead, the booze was watered down, and Ralph, noting that the band now outnumbered the patrons, was bone tired and had a headache. Not to mention that for the last few days his hands had felt as if they had molasses circulating through them. He'd played almost every slow tune he knew earlier in the evening, but things hadn't loosened up much. Now his hands were starting to ache. Even his hair hurt, he thought.

When he got home, he fell into bed and immediately went to sleep. But later that morning (actually, more like noon), Ralph regained consciousness, stumbled into the bathroom, and tried to turn on the shower faucet. To his surprise, he found that he could not grip it well enough to twist it to the right. Then he took a closer look at his hands. The thumb

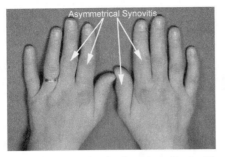

Figure 6-1: Hands of a female patient with psoriatic arthritis, distributed asymmetrically, like Ralph's arthritis.

and index fingers of the right hand and the index and middle fingers of the left hand were swollen up like sausages.

Both of his hands were so stiff that he could hardly move them, and when he tried, his hands felt as though they had been crushed in a car door. This situation was not compatible with the demands of his profession. He had read about the brilliant concert pianist Leon Fleisher, who at the peak of his skills had lost the use of his right hand. At least Fleisher, whose problem was not arthritic, always had the use of his left hand, and for many years he was able to make something of a career out of playing Ravel's Piano Concerto for Left Hand, but both of Ralph's hands were out of commission. Ralph also knew that Fleisher eventually (after nearly 40 years) regained the use of his right hand, and he was determined to seek treatment for his problem immediately. He called his doctor's office and set up a visit for the next day.

Ralph's Assessment

Ralph described his problems and his worries about potential disability to the doctor, a family-practice physician who asked him a few questions and examined him briefly. Then he escorted Ralph down the hall to a rheumatologist's office.

After the rheumatologist examined Ralph, among the first questions he asked were how long Ralph's scalp had been bothering him and whether he had any other skin problems. Ralph responded that he had some itchiness in the ears and that he had noted some scaling over the knees and elbows. The rheumatologist then ordered some laboratory tests and X-rays. Before Ralph left the office to get the testing done, the doctor said, "Ralph, the good news is that you don't have what Leon Fleisher had. The bad news is that I think you have psoriasis complicated by one of the common forms of arthritis that can accompany this skin disease. We'll confirm that you have psoriatic arthritis by ruling out other forms of arthritis and then get you going on a treatment program. In the meantime, let's start you on an anti-inflammatory medication to try to make you a little more comfortable." He gave Ralph a prescription for sulindac, 200 milligrams twice daily, to be taken with food, and sent him on his way.

Ralph returned to the rheumatologist's office the following week, having had blood tests and X-rays of his hands and wrists. He was feeling slightly improved on the sulindac but was hoping to get a lot more relief. The doctor went over the results with him, explaining that the X-rays showed evidence only of soft-tissue swelling around the joints of Ralph's swollen fingers. There was no sign of joint damage. Meanwhile, the blood tests revealed only an elevated erythrocyte sedimentation rate, confirmation of active inflammation.

All about Psoriatic Arthritis

What causes psoriatic arthritis?

The cause(s) of psoriasis and psoriatic arthritis remain(s) unknown.

What are the symptoms of psoriatic arthritis?

As with all forms of inflammatory arthritis, psoriatic arthritis presents with painful swelling and stiffness of the involved joints. Usually the arthritis does not appear until some time after the onset of skin involvement, but there are cases in which the arthritis begins first. In these situations, the diagnosis may be difficult until the skin manifestations appear. Psoriatic arthritis can take any of five main forms.

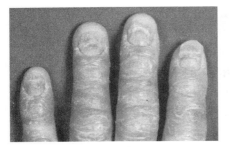

Figure 6-2: Hand of a patient with highly active psoriasis and arthritis attacking the DIP (distal interphalangeal) joints. Note the damage to the fingernails, typical of this form of psoriatic arthritis.

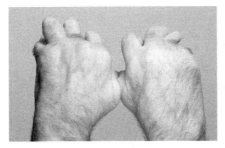

Figure 6-3: Hands of a patient with the most destructive form of psoriatic arthritis, called arthritis mutilans, for obvious reasons.

One type affects the outermost joints of the fingers—the distal interphalangeal, or DIP, joints—which become swollen and quite painful.

In this form, the nails usually become pitted or pull away from the underlying nail beds. If the skin involvement is not obvious, this can be easily mistaken for osteoarthritis of the hands.

A second type involves mainly the spine and closely resembles ankylosing spondylitis (described in chapter 5). This psoriatic spondylitis is usually accompanied by a positive blood test for the HLA-B27 antigen. Ralph wasn't even tested for B27 because, based on his symptoms, he clearly didn't have spondylitis.

The third version, which is what Ralph had, is characterized by involvement of just a few joints—called oligoarticular—usually with an asymmetrical distribution. That is, the same joints are not affected on both sides. The disease may or may not be destructive, but if it remains active, the risk of joint destruction is certainly greater.

Type four looks just like rheumatoid arthritis, in that it is symmetrical and seropositive for rheumatoid factor); it may represent the co-occurrence of two common diseases—rheumatoid arthritis and psoriasis—rather than a special form of psoriatic arthritis.

The fifth type is very destructive and goes by the ominous name of arthritis mutilans.

What tests do I need?

If you suspect that you have psoriatic arthritis, you will want to have a blood test and X-rays performed. Like Ralph, if you have psoriatic arthritis, your X-rays will reveal only soft tissue inflammation around the joints unless there is damage to the joint itself, in which case your physician will see evidence of damage, such as erosions, on the film. Your blood test results will likely show an elevated sedimentation rate.

When you have active inflammation, your body produces blood proteins that cause red blood cells (erythrocytes) to stick together and settle, or sediment, more rapidly than normal. This is measured in a special narrow glass tube, and the rate at which the cells settle is called the sedimentation rate. An elevated sedimentation rate is a very nonspecific test and suggests only that there is inflammation somewhere in your body. It is elevated in many different forms of arthritis, not only in psoriatic arthritis. Sometimes successful treatment makes the sedimentation rate return toward normal, and it is used as a rough indicator of the activity of the process.

As with Ralph, if all your other tests are normal or negative, that is consistent with the diagnosis of psoriatic arthritis—provided, of course, that you definitely have psoriasis. As previously noted, psoriatic lesions may not be present at the onset of arthritis. The skin abnormalities Ralph's doctor observed had the typical appearance of psoriasis, and they were located in several of the usual places: the scalp, the ear canals, and over the knees and elbows.

Is psoriasis milder in people with psoriatic arthritis?

Not necessarily. The skin rash of psoriasis can be of any degree of severity in psoriatic arthritis, and it does not tend to fluctuate relative to the activity of the arthritis. The relationship between what is going on with the skin and joint activity is complex and not always apparent.

Is psoriatic arthritis genetic?

There is evidence that susceptibility to psoriasis and psoriatic arthritis is inherited. Attempts to localize the gene(s) involved have produced conflicting results, but several research groups are working on this issue.

Does psoriatic arthritis predispose me to other diseases?

Psoriatic arthritis is really just a type of arthritis that commonly presents in patients with the skin disease psoriasis. But there are at least three other kinds of arthritis that may occur in association with psoriasis: rheumatoid arthritis, gouty arthritis, and sarcoid arthritis.

Rheumatoid arthritis Both psoriasis and rheumatoid arthritis are common, and it stands to reason that unless one protects against the other—which does not seem to be the case—both would occasionally be present in the same person. Ralph's doctor ruled out rheumatoid arthritis for a couple of reasons. First, Ralph's arthritis was asymmetrical, and rheumatoid arthritis is usually symmetrical. Moreover, his rheumatoid factor test was negative. Rheumatoid factor is an antibody that reacts with a normal blood protein called IgG. About 80 percent of people with rheumatoid arthritis, including those who also have psoriasis, test positive for rheumatoid factor; that is, they are seropositive.

Gouty arthritis Gout is fairly common in people with psoriasis, particularly if the psoriasis is very widely distributed and actively spreading. This probably occurs because in active psoriasis there is rapid cellular turnover in the involved skin, resulting in the generation of a lot of cellular breakdown substances, including uric acid. When the uric acid concentration in the blood and body fluids, including joint fluid, is high, it tends to crystallize as sodium urate in the joints, causing attacks of gouty arthritis.

Ralph's psoriasis was neither widespread nor particularly active, and his uric acid level was normal. Although gout rarely presents as an asymmetrical arthritis affecting a few joints, the most common picture is inflammation of a single joint. If there were any doubt, the doctor could have aspirated some fluid from one of Ralph's finger joints and looked for sodium urate crystals, but this seemed so unlikely that he decided to spare Ralph that procedure.

Sarcoid arthritis Sarcoidosis is another inflammatory disease that occurs a little more frequently in people with psoriasis than in the population at large. Although sarcoidosis usually attacks the lungs, once in a while men and women with this disease exhibit involvement of other organ systems, including the joints. This can take the form of an arthritic condition affecting multiple joints. Ralph did not have any other signs of sarcoidosis, such as abnormalities in the chest X-ray, enlarged lymph nodes, spleen, and/or salivary glands, and typical findings of sarcoid arthritis on the joint X-rays. Therefore the doctor concluded that his arthritis was not due to sarcoidosis.

Can psoriatic arthritis be prevented?

There is no known way to effectively prevent psoriatic arthritis.

Can diet help?

Dietary measures are not known to be helpful in psoriatic arthritis.

Should I exercise if I have psoriatic arthritis?

The same principles of exercise and physical therapy that apply in rheumatoid arthritis apply to psoriatic arthritis. Generally, if you are diagnosed with psoriatic arthritis you should avoid high-impact exercises such as running. Walking is a good alternative, and swimming is even better. It's important for you to follow an exercise program designed by a physical medicine expert, such as a physiatrist or a physical or occupational therapist, in order to minimize the likelihood of causing damage to joints and tendons.

How common is psoriatic arthritis?

Although many people haven't heard of it, psoriatic arthritis is fairly common. No reliable statistics are available.

Treating Psoriatic Arthritis

The drug treatment, surgical treatment, and physical rehabilitation treatment for psoriatic arthritis are similar to those recommended for rheumatoid arthritis. Care must be exercised in the use of corticosteroids and antimalarial drugs, both of which have been associated with a serious but uncommon complication of psoriasis known as pustular psoriasis. Nevertheless, we frequently use these drugs to treat severe psoriatic arthritis, and untoward effects are rare. Biological agents such as the anti-TNF-alpha inhibitors are becoming more widely used with good results. The same caveats about the possible long-term side effects of these agents apply.

Can psoriatic arthritis be cured?

There is no cure for psoriatic arthritis.

What factors are considered when choosing a treatment plan?

The considerations are the same as in rheumatoid arthritis. Ralph's doctor started with an NSAID, planning to add hydroxychloroquine and methotrexate later if needed. Methotrexate and hydroxychloroquine belong to the category of DMARDs, which stands for disease-modifying antirheumatic drugs. These drugs can modify the course of psoriatic arthritis in some patients, delaying and perhaps preventing erosion of the affected joints. Methotrexate has the additional advantage in patients with psoriatic arthritis of improving the skin manifestations of psoriasis as well.

The doctor considered starting Ralph on a low dose of prednisone, too. Prednisone is a synthetic cortisone-like drug that has been available for many years. It works fast and provides symptomatic relief, at least initially, for most patients. He ultimately decided against this as a first-line approach because of the drug's side effects over time, especially its tendency to cause osteoporosis, even in low doses. Once started, prednisone is very difficult to discontinue because it suppresses the body's ability to make its own cortisone.

Ralph's Treatment

The rheumatologist had immediately started Ralph on the nonsteroidal anti-inflammatory sulindac. By the time Ralph returned for the results of his test, he'd been taking the full dosage for about a week, which gave the doctor a good idea of how well things would go with that drug as the sole treatment. Judging from Ralph's insignificant response, patient and doctor agreed that sulindac alone wasn't going to do the trick.

Sulindac belongs to the drug class known as nonsteroidal (meaning not cortisone-like) anti-inflammatory drugs. Such drugs are more simply called NSAIDs (pronounced EN-seds). The most familiar NSAID is aspirin. There are a number of nonsteroidal anti-inflammatories, and different people react differently to them. In any given person, it is impossible to say up front which drug would be the best.

Because the treatment for psoriatic arthritis is similar to that for rheumatoid arthritis, Ralph's doctor noted that they could try each of the NSAIDs, one after the other, to see which one worked best for Ralph. However, given the minimal response that he got with sulindac, it seemed unlikely, even if there was one that worked better, that an NSAID would produce a completely satisfactory result. Furthermore, it would take several months to give each of the NSAIDs a fair trial, and neither Ralph nor the doctor wanted to delay more effective treatment that long.

Medication

Ralph's doctor advocated moving to the next step on the treatment ladder: methotrexate. He skipped the antimalarial hydroxychloroquine to avoid the previously mentioned small risk of producing pustular psoriasis, a serious complication of psoriasis. Although methotrexate is a form of chemotherapy, with careful monitoring it's pretty safe, as drugs for arthritis go, especially in the relatively low doses used in psoriatic arthritis. It has also been proven effective in treating psoriasis, but the dosages required to clear up psoriatic skin lesions are much higher than those needed to treat the joints. Ralph's relatively minimal amount of skin involvement didn't warrant this high-dose treatment.

The doctor prescribed Ralph five tablets of methotrexate—a total dose of 12.5 milligrams—each Monday, and directed him to continue taking the sulindac. On such a regimen, you can expect to see some improvement in your arthritis symptoms in four to six weeks. The improvement may occur so gradually that you will not notice it unless you think back to how you felt when you started. Depending on how you are doing after a couple of months, your doctor may consider additional treatment.

Ralph was asked to return for follow-up visits at two-month intervals so that his doctor could check his response to the medications and make sure that he was showing adequate improvement. He also wanted to monitor Ralph to make sure he wasn't having any side effects.

Ralph's Response to Treatment

For a couple of weeks after starting methotrexate, Ralph couldn't detect any significant change in his condition, but he stuck with it; he wasn't getting worse, and there was nothing to suggest the medicine was causing problems for him. He resolved that he would persevere until the first follow-up visit unless things got materially worse. He did, and they didn't.

During this time, he continued to work. Although he didn't feel great, he could still get around the keyboard. He developed an introspective, economical playing style, more like that of the Modern Jazz Quartet's John Lewis than that of his previous model, the flamboyant Oscar Peterson. He found the change to be intellectually challenging, and Arlo, his bass player, got into the spirit of things as well, embracing the new fuguelike style. Even the drummer, Freddy, occasionally mustered what passed for a smile in his limited repertoire of facial expressions, but mostly he just grunted now and then and stared glassily into the great unknown as he brushed his drums.

As time passed, Ralph increasingly played for hours without even thinking about his arthritis.

First follow-up visit

The two months were up. Time for Ralph's first follow-up visit with the rheumatologist. Although he was still having mild swelling and stiffness in several fingers, he had clearly improved. The doctor was impressed with his progress and his success in adapting to the limitations imposed by his condition. But several finger joints were still swollen. Ralph's skin condition hadn't improved either, though it hadn't worsened.

Ralph's blood count and liver function tests were normal, and there was no evidence of methotrexate toxicity. But his doctor was concerned that the arthritis was only partially controlled. As with any arthritic condition, uncontrolled psoriatic arthritis can lead to joint damage over time.

What happens if treatment stops working?

Ralph and his doctor determined that the best course of action was to continue the present treatment and see what happened. However, the rheumatologist explained that in the future, especially if things didn't go well, he might recommend that Ralph try one of the TNF-alpha inhibitors.

TNF-alpha inhibitors A growing literature suggests that these drugs are useful in patients with various forms of inflammatory arthritis, including psoriatic arthritis. Currently, three such drugs are available: etanercept, infliximab, and adalimumab.

"Tell me more about this TNF-alpha," Ralph inquired. "How well can I expect this to work? Are there any hazards to this treatment?"

The doctor answered by saying that although the short-term hazards of using these drugs seem acceptable, we really don't know what problems they may cause after years of use. They do predispose people to infections, and these are sometimes serious, but they can usually be treated successfully with antibiotics and by temporarily withdrawing the TNF-alpha inhibitor. Nevertheless, the biggest worry is that they may predispose a person to developing certain kinds of malignant tumors; for example, lymphomas, which are difficult to treat. Infliximab already seems to be generating lymphomas. We don't know how frequently this may occur, and that will become clearer with time. What we do know is that these drugs often work very well in people with arthritis, and in psoriatic arthritis they may clear the skin lesions as well. One side effect, recently described, is hives, but this doesn't occur very often.

What to Expect

Psoriasis is an incurable, chronic relapsing disease affecting the skin and, in many cases, the joints as well. Typically, the disease may present

Disease at a Glance: Psoriatic Arthritis

Who Gets It?

- People who have had psoriasis for five to ten years (but in a few, the arthritis comes before the rash)
- Males and females equally affected
- Frequent family history

Joint Involvement

- Five overlapping types:
  - DIP joints with nail changes (10 percent)
  - Rheumatoid arthritis–like distribution (25 percent)
  - Oligoarticular, asymmetrical (80 percent)
  - Spondylitislike (5 to 20 percent)
  - Mutilans (uncommon)
- Destructive, erosive
- Sausage-like swelling of involved joints

Other Features and Complications

- Psoriasis, usually with nail changes
- Gout
- Sarcoidosis

Lab Results

- Elevated acute-phase reactants (sedimentation rate and C-reactive protein)
- Rheumatoid factor usually negative (except for the rheumatoid arthritis–like type)

Treatment

- General
  - Adequate rest
  - Appropriate exercise
  - Education

(continued)

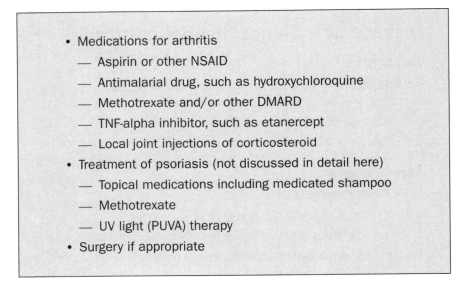

- Medications for arthritis
  — Aspirin or other NSAID
  — Antimalarial drug, such as hydroxychloroquine
  — Methotrexate and/or other DMARD
  — TNF-alpha inhibitor, such as etanercept
  — Local joint injections of corticosteroid
- Treatment of psoriasis (not discussed in detail here)
  — Topical medications including medicated shampoo
  — Methotrexate
  — UV light (PUVA) therapy
- Surgery if appropriate

differently in the skin than it does in the joints; therefore it usually becomes necessary to treat each aspect of the disease somewhat independently. Since there is a real possibility of joint destruction leading to disability in psoriatic arthritis, it is important to treat the arthritis aggressively, using the methods outlined in this chapter.

Will I be disabled?

In the great majority of people with psoriatic arthritis, the disease can be controlled well enough that they can carry on their daily activities pretty much as they did before, especially if it is caught early. Fortunately, the new treatments are more effective than the previous ones we had, so our success rate in dealing with this disease should continue to improve.

Nevertheless, in some people psoriatic arthritis can be quite destructive, in much the same manner as rheumatoid arthritis. If the inflammatory process cannot be controlled, localized damage to cartilage and bone can occur, leading to permanently reduced mobility and to deformity of the involved joints—even to fusion of the joints.

Ralph's Outcome

As the months went by, Ralph's improvement continued. His career took off as well, and over the next few years he did not have any significant recurrences of his arthritis. He continued to sit for blood tests several times a year to check for evidence of methotrexate toxicity. On one occasion, he developed a painful mouth ulcer. His doctor lowered his dose and added a weekly dose of folic acid, a B vitamin that reduces the drug's toxic effects, and the ulcer cleared. Ralph moved to California, where the weather was more to his liking and where his recording company was based.

Chapter 7

Adult Still's Disease and Juvenile Chronic Polyarthritis

Onset: I've Got the Fever!

It was summer, but uncharacteristically, Earlene was feeling poorly. She was 28 years old but felt as if she were 80. This was all the more surprising to her in light of the fact that she always kept herself physically fit through eating right, getting plenty of rest, and exercising religiously. She had to because of her job as a guard in the county detention center. She took pride in the fact that under normal circumstances there were no other women and only a few men—either inmates or fellow guards—whom she could not disable instantaneously with a well-placed kick and a takedown. She was voluptuously good-looking, and several adventurous males had discovered her self-defense skills for

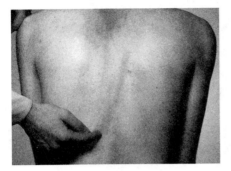

Figure 7-1: Koebner's phenomenon in a patient with adult-onset Still's disease. Note the broad area of reaction to a light scratch by the physician.

themselves. Word had spread, and it was rare that anybody tried anything with her these days.

Today was bad, though. Although this was the fifth time that she had felt this way over the past three months, this episode was definitely the worst. Each spell had lasted several days, with the symptoms coming and going once or twice a day. Today it was hard work just to walk down the hall.

She felt alternately hot and cold. She was stiff, and her joints were sore. Her hands were diffusely swollen. Earlene noticed a subtle, slightly raised, splotchy rash widely scattered over her body. It didn't itch, but when she ran a long, carefully tended fingernail over her skin, she was surprised to see a welt gradually arise in its path. Her throat felt sore. She was a mess.

Earlene headed for the infirmary to see whether she could get some aspirin and was pleased to see that her running pal Gladys was the duty nurse.

She sat down, and Gladys stuck a thermometer into her mouth. After a few minutes, Gladys removed the thermometer, looked at it, raised her eyebrows, and gave a low whistle. "A hundred and three! Now that's something." She placed a tongue blade into Earlene's mouth, turned on a flashlight, and peered down her friend's throat. It was red but otherwise looked pretty normal.

Gladys took her hand and squeezed it lightly, unintentionally shooting a bolt of pain through Earlene's wrist and forearm. "Yikes, woman, take it easy!" yelped Earlene. "I appreciate the thought, but you don't have to break my hand!" Earlene was about to ask the nurse to examine her skin, but when she looked again, she was amazed that in the few minutes since she had come into the infirmary, the rash had disappeared.

Concerned, Gladys picked up the phone and rang the "doctor" on call. Third- and fourth-year medical students, living and working as externs at the county home for the elderly across the street, took first call at the detention center. A half hour later, a tired-looking young man presented himself in the infirmary and introduced himself as Oscar, the doctor on call.

Earlene told him her story, and Oscar listened attentively, making some notes on the chart as she talked. When she finished, he asked her a few questions about her past medical history and especially her family medical history. He asked if she had been around anybody with an infectious illness, to which she replied in the negative. In the review of systems (the part of the medical history in which the physician asks a series of specific questions pertaining to every system of the body: circulatory, neurological, and so forth), Oscar asked Earlene if she was sexually active, to which she replied, "Whenever possible." She replied negatively when he asked her about a vaginal discharge.

By this time, Earlene was beginning to feel a little better. When Oscar took her temperature, it had returned to normal and her throat didn't feel quite as bad. Still, the doctor began a systematic examination. Aside from some redness in the back of her throat and tenderness in the small joints of her hands and wrists, there was not much to find. He confirmed that scratching the skin resulted in the formation of a welt. He was very careful to ascertain that Earlene's spleen was not enlarged, and that there were no enlarged lymph nodes in the neck, armpits, or groin areas, or around the elbows or knees, which might have suggested infection or leukemia.

"Okay," said Oscar, "I think we're pretty much done here. Why don't you go ahead and get dressed, and then we'll talk about this."

Earlene's Assessment

The doctor gave Earlene a working diagnosis: a rare condition called adult Still's disease. Still's disease is an arthritic condition that usually affects very young children. The symptoms are swollen painful joints, high fever, a salmon-colored fleeting rash—one that comes and goes quickly, even within a few minutes—sometimes a sore throat, and in many cases a peculiar skin reaction known as Koebner's phenomenon (the appearance of welts with light scratching of the skin). He ordered some tests in order to gather more information.

A few days later, Earlene returned to the infirmary to get her report. Somewhat to her surprise, standing next to Oscar and Gladys was a portly, elderly gentleman whom Oscar introduced as his physician preceptor, a rheumatologist of some local repute who was there to supervise the proceedings. After the introductions, the rheumatologist said that Oscar's original working diagnosis appeared to be correct and that Earlene, indeed, had adult Still's disease.

All about Adult Still's Disease

Sir George F. Still was a British pediatrician whose life spanned the last third of the 19th century and the first half of the 20th. The disease is named after him because he provided the first written description of 22 cases of it in his M.D. thesis in 1896. He described what he called "a chronic joint disease in children." Ten years later he became the first chairman of a hospital pediatrics department in England, and in his later years, he served as the pediatrician to the royal family, caring for the young princesses Elizabeth and Margaret.

The arthritis of Still's disease affects multiple joints and may be mild or severe. Although Still referred to the disease as chronic, it isn't always, sometimes entering complete remission with no recurrence. When it is chronic, there tends to be destruction of the affected joints unless it is treated aggressively.

Adult Still's disease presents doctors with a special challenge because there is no lab test to confirm the diagnosis. In a way, this is a diagnosis of exclusion: if we can exclude all the other possibilities, then it has to be adult-onset Still's disease.

Certain infections could cause the symptoms Earlene described, such as gonorrhea and meningococcemia, a bloodstream infection with the germ responsible for bacterial meningitis, but there are others as well. However, these were ruled out because Earlene did not have a vaginal discharge and the blood cultures were sterile. AIDS was also eliminated by the lab tests. Rheumatic fever, an autoimmune disease often affecting the heart valves, caused by certain types of streptococcus could also do it, but the throat culture was negative for streptococcus—the cause of rheumatic fever—and the rash wasn't typical. Systemic lupus erythematosus is another autoimmune disease that can produce similar symptoms, but the lab tests for lupus were negative, and the distribution of the rash wasn't confined to sun-exposed areas of skin as in lupus. Occasionally, certain forms of leukemia can also start this way. Again, the lab tests ruled this out, as did the fact that Earlene didn't have an enlarged spleen or lymph nodes. The fleeting nature of her symptoms was more suggestive of adult-onset Still's disease than anything else.

What causes adult Still's disease?

The cause of Still's disease, whether it starts in infancy, childhood, or adulthood, is unknown. This is, in fact, true of most forms of arthritis. Theories range from infection to autoimmunity, but there is little or no support for any of these possible mechanisms. In fact, although adult and juvenile Still's disease look alike clinically (except, of course, for the age of the patient), we can't really be certain that they are one and the same disease or even that all childhood or all adult cases of Still's disease have the same cause. For practical purposes we assume they're the same because they act alike, but we really don't know for sure.

What are the symptoms of adult Still's disease?

Still's disease is an arthritic condition with bouts of fever, often quite high; a fleeting, recurrent, salmon-colored rash; sore throat; and sometimes other symptoms. The fever often has a pattern of one or two peaks daily, up to 103 degrees, with periods of relatively

Earlene's doctors were pretty certain that she was suffering from adult Still's disease, but there are other diseases that also produce fever, rash, and arthritis. When the symptoms a person experiences could indicate any number of diseases, the list of possible culprits is called the differential diagnosis. Figuring out which item on the differential diagnosis is causing the symptoms is a form of medical detective work. Physicians enjoy the intellectual challenge of figuring out the real diagnosis by looking at the differential diagnosis and narrowing the list.

normal temperature in between. The rash tends to be most prominent when the temperature is highest, and it may clear completely between fever spikes. The arthritis affects multiple joints.

What is Koebner's phenomenon?

Oscar had also observed that Earlene exhibited Koebner's phenomenon. Heinrich Koebner—usually pronounced KEB-ner by English speakers, and originally spelled Köbner—was a German skin doctor, and he practically founded the specialty of dermatology in Breslau, Germany, which is now in Poland and goes by the name of Wroclaw. He was born about 30 years before Still and died just after the beginning of the 20th century. His most famous accomplishment is that he noticed and described a phenomenon that occurs in psoriasis and certain other diseases, in which mechanical irritation of the skin, such as a scratch, provokes a reaction at the site of the irritation that he called an isomorphic reaction. People liked the term Koebner's phenomenon better, and that is what it is called today in memory of old Heinrich. This reaction to mechanical stimulation is common in Still's disease.

How does Still's disease fit into the spectrum of arthritis?

Though Still's disease typically afflicts children, adults can have Still's disease in two different ways. Still's disease can be chronic, starting in childhood and persisting into adulthood, although in many cases it goes into a permanent remission. However, the condition we typically call adult Still's disease begins in adulthood and therefore might more correctly be referred to as adult-onset Still's disease. Since the cause is unknown, and the reason for the relationship to childhood is not clear, we probably shouldn't be too surprised that it can manifest in adults. But diseases that begin in unusual ways, especially rare ones, are harder to diagnose because physicians usually don't think of them in that context.

In children, Still's disease is one of the four common forms of arthritis, the other three being oligoarticular or pauciarticular (both words meaning "few joints"); juvenile chronic arthritis; and polyarticular adult-form rheumatoid arthritis presenting in childhood. The latter behaves just like rheumatoid arthritis in adults, and it often continues into adulthood.

The oligoarticular form of juvenile arthritis involves only a few joints, and these are typically distributed asymmetrically—that is, a finger joint or two on one hand and a wrist on the opposite side, or any other combination of two to four joints. This form of arthritis occurs almost exclusively in girls, and it is often accompanied by eye inflammation that can lead to blindness if not recognized and treated aggressively. About 60 percent of these patients eventually go into a permanent remission. Those that don't eventually become another group of adults with juvenile-onset arthritis.

Is adult Still's disease genetic?

Adult Still's disease is so rare that more than one case in a family is almost never observed, so it doesn't run in families, as it were. Nevertheless, a considerable amount of evidence suggests that juvenile arthritis has a hereditary or genetic component, but the focus of these studies has not for the most part been on Still's disease per se. In Still's disease, genetically determined abnormalities have been described in certain chemical mediators of inflammation, but not all investigators have confirmed these.

Most recently, a group of Japanese scientists found evidence of a high-level association of a genetically determined abnormality on a mediator protein called interleukin-18 (IL-18) in people with adult Still's disease. They also found IL-18 to be present in higher than normal concentrations in people with adult Still's disease. If that research holds up to further scrutiny by other labs, it could well be the first direct genetic link in the disease. The short answer, though, is that we don't know for sure as yet.

Does adult Still's disease predispose me to other diseases?

The answer to this question is not known.

Can adult Still's disease be prevented?

There is no known way to prevent this rare disease or even to identify people at risk for developing it.

Does diet help?

Diet is not known to affect the disease.

Should I exercise if I have adult Still's disease?

As previously noted, one of the biggest problems for people with arthritis, whether it is rheumatoid or some other form, is that painful joints tend to make you less active. However, avoiding exercise and physical activity in general begins a vicious cycle: the inactivity leads to muscle wasting, which in turn leads to decreased strength and even less activity, until a person becomes completely disabled. Inactivity also promotes weight gain, another big problem for all the obvious health reasons as well as the extra burden on arthritic, weight-bearing joints.

On the other hand, certain kinds of activity can be destructive to joints that may already have some damage from arthritis. Generally, if you are diagnosed with adult Still's disease with chronic arthritis, you should avoid high-impact exercises such as running. Walking is a good alternative, and swimming is even better. It's important for you to follow an exercise program designed by a physical medicine expert, such as a physiatrist or a physical or occupational therapist, in order to minimize the likelihood of causing damage to joints and tendons.

How common is adult Still's disease?

Adult Still's disease is quite rare, occurring in less than 0.1 percent of the population.

Treating Adult Still's Disease

There really aren't enough cases of adult Still's disease to make scientifically sound clinical trials of potential therapies practical. Although adult Still's disease and rheumatoid arthritis differ in many respects, we tend to treat them alike. They are both inflammatory diseases of unknown cause, and both target the joints. Both conditions can damage joints; therefore it is important to bring them under control before they lead to disability.

We know from experience that the old "go low, go slow" approach—that is, start with low doses of medications and escalate only after an adequate trial of the least dangerous and least effective drugs, such as aspirin—eventually brings the disease under some semblance of control in many patients, but a lot of joint damage can occur while we are slowly getting there. It's better to start more aggressively with more powerful drugs (see below).

Can adult Still's disease be cured?

There is no known cure for adult Still's disease, but some cases go into spontaneous remission, as previously noted.

What factors are considered when choosing a treatment plan?

The same principles that govern treatment selection in rheumatoid arthritis (see chapter 2) apply to adult Still's disease.

Earlene's Treatment

Medication

Earlene's doctor recommended that she start with a moderately aggressive combination of four types of oral medication (see chapter 2 for the details of administration and a discussion of possible side effects):

- Nonsteroidal anti-inflammatory drug (naproxen)
- Antimalarial drug (hydroxychloroquine)
- Antimetabolite (methotrexate)
- Corticosteroid (prednisone)

Prednisone, taken initially in moderately high dosage—20 to 40 milligrams daily—usually brings the fever down in a hurry and gets rid of the rash, while the others work more slowly, especially hydroxychloroquine and methotrexate. But Earlene's doctor wanted to start all the drugs at the same time, then withdraw the prednisone during the early phase of treatment.

He gave her several prescriptions, including naproxen, 375 milligrams twice daily with food; hydroxychloroquine, 200 milligrams twice daily; methotrexate, 12.5 milligrams once weekly; and prednisone, 30 milligrams once daily. If the disease continued to recur, he told her, they would consider using the more potent new biological therapies, such as a TNF-alpha inhibitor. There is also some evidence that anakinra, an inhibitor of interleukin-1 (IL-1), a mediator of inflammation similar to TNF-alpha, may be effective and may even be the biological agent of choice in Still's disease.

What are the side effects of this treatment?

Every drug has side effects, and the drugs used to treat adult Still's disease are quite potent, so the possibility of experiencing side effects is significant. For example, prednisone works rapidly and is likely to improve your arthritis within a few hours. But if you continue at this dose for more than a few days, you'll begin to see evidence of side effects. It is a strong appetite stimulant, and you will eat more and gain weight rapidly. The weight gain is associated with a characteristic distribution of body fat to the face and trunk but not to the limbs. It also causes thinning of the skin and easy bruising, particularly on the arms and legs. In addition, prednisone can cause a form of diabetes—high blood sugar and impaired sugar metabolism—and it can lead to osteoporosis; that is, thinning and softening of bone, resulting in fractures and curvature of the spine. It also causes acne. Many people who take this amount of predni-sone feel euphoric and energized, even to the point that they have difficulty sleeping at night.

Naproxen, a commonly used nonsteroidal anti-inflammatory drug, should begin working within a day but may not reach full potency for several days or even a couple of weeks. The most common side effect of naproxen is upset stomach, but over time the drug can cause peptic ulcers in the stomach or small intestine. Less frequently, it can cause impaired kidney function, hypertension, liver damage, and ringing of the ears with hearing loss. Interestingly, after several decades of use, new data suggests that this drug may be associated with an increase in the frequency of heart attacks. This finding comes on the heels of a number of reports of similar problems with the selective COX-2-inhibiting NSAIDs. It is surprising in view of the fact that naproxen is a nonselective NSAID that inhibits both COX-1 and COX-2 and that the drug has been around so long without any hint of such a problem.

Hydroxychloroquine works considerably more slowly, usually requiring 8 to 12 weeks to reach full potency. The most common side effects occur in the gastrointestinal tract and can vary from flatulence to nausea and vomiting. The most treacherous side effects are in the eyes and in the worst-case scenario can lead to blindness. When you are taking hydroxychloroquine, your doctor will want to schedule annual eye examinations. The following problems can arise, but are rare: skin rash, weakness, enlargement of the heart (cardiomyopathy) and heart failure, and a blood disorder in people lacking the enzyme glucose-6-phosphate dehydrogenase.

Methotrexate works by inhibiting the body's ability to use folic acid. The B vitamin is needed to form DNA, the most important building block for genes, required for cell reproduction. Since in active inflammation, inflammatory cells must reproduce rapidly, methotrexate inhibits inflammation by slowing this process. It also has an inhibitory effect on other parts of the body where cells reproduce rapidly, including the bone marrow—where blood cells are formed—and the liver. This is the basis for the main side effects of methotrexate: low levels of red blood cells, white blood cells, and/or platelets, and liver damage. These effects are reversible by stopping the drug. Methotrexate can also have other side effects, such as nausea and vomiting, menstrual irregularities, and drowsiness. Pregnant women or those trying to get pregnant should not take it. Methotrexate takes several weeks to reach its full effectiveness, but generally by 12 weeks we can tell how well it is going to work for you.

Can I have children while taking these medications?

Methotrexate reduces fertility, but if a woman should happen to become pregnant while taking it or starts it while already pregnant, continued use of methotrexate often leads to a miscarriage. Furthermore, because of the way methotrexate works, its presence in the mother's body during the early stages of pregnancy could lead to deformities in the developing baby. It's best to simply avoid getting pregnant while on methotrexate.

Earlene's Response to Treatment

Earlene filled the prescriptions on her way home from work that Friday evening and began taking them the next morning. The first change she noticed was that by late Saturday afternoon she felt euphoric: full of energy and eager to clean out the garage and the attic. She felt more like a 28-year-old ought to feel, in her estimation. In addition, her appetite was voracious. She usually got together with Gladys on Saturday night and shared a pizza for dinner. That evening she consumed (inhaled is more like it) three-quarters of a 12-slice pepperoni pizza.

After Gladys went home, Earlene cleaned up the mess and went to bed, but she couldn't sleep. Her mind was racing, pondering all the things she was going to do the next day and throughout the coming week. Finally she gave up, turned on her lamp, and tried to read. Her taste ran to steamy novels, and she was working on a real barn-burner. Alas, it was no good; even the purple, athletic prose to which she was so addicted couldn't keep her attention. She called her boyfriend, Fred, but he wasn't at home, or at least wasn't answering his phone. She got up, poured herself a glass of merlot, filled the bathtub with hot water, and slipped in for a relaxing soak. After the bath and the third glass of merlot, she began to feel a little drowsy. Around two o'clock in the morning, she finally fell asleep.

The next day, Earlene's joints were less painful, and she continued to feel as though she were running on jet fuel. Fred was finally home from a short business trip, and he came over to see what was going on. As soon as he walked in the door, she was all over him, and before he knew it they were having passionate sex with Earlene as the aggressor. Fred was surprised but flattered as well. As he regained his composure, he asked her, "What did that doctor do to you? I definitely like it!"

First follow-up visit and subsequent course of treatment

At the end of the week, Fred was really tired, but Earlene was still going strong. At the office, the rheumatologist greeted them cordially.

"How are you feeling, Earlene?" he asked.

"My joints have never felt better!" she chirped. "My fever is gone, and the rash hasn't come back either. In fact, I feel great!"

But Fred had another side of the story to tell. He reported that Earlene was eating five times as much as she used to. She wasn't getting much sleep, either—her energy was so high that she was running him ragged! And though initially thrilled at her surge of sexual interest, Fred explained somewhat sheepishly that he couldn't keep up with her.

The doctor could tell right away that Earlene was experiencing prednisone-induced euphoria. He relayed to Fred the treatment plan he had outlined for Earlene the week before, including the side effects of the drugs, focusing especially on prednisone and hydroxychloroquine. Fred listened attentively and calmed down considerably.

Though Earlene's arthritis was being controlled mainly by prednisone (and, to a lesser extent, naproxen, since the other drugs hadn't taken effect yet), the doctor was concerned that she was beginning to have side effects mainly from the prednisone. He elected to reduce the dose. He'd been prepared to do this anyway, even in the absence of side effects, assuming that the disease had settled down, which it clearly had.

The doctor then outlined a plan for gradual prednisone reduction to a more tolerable dose of 5 milligrams daily over a one-month period, while continuing the other medications. During this time, Earlene's personality, energy level, and (to Fred's relief) appetites returned to normal, and over the next 12 months, the arthritis and other symptoms of Still's disease remained quiet, apparently controlled by the combination of hydroxychloroquine, naproxen, low-dose prednisone, and methotrexate. Although Earlene had a little increased flatulence, no other side effects were apparent, and she was able to work regularly and resume her previous life.

About a year after the initial episode of illness, Earlene began to notice some swelling and stiffness in the small joints of her hands and wrists. At first these symptoms were intermittent, but they became more constant over the next couple of months and began to be accompanied by a lot of pain. She had no fever or rash. The doctor advised her to increase the methotrexate to 15 milligrams per week, but this really didn't provide much relief.

What happens if treatment stops working?

At the next visit, the doctor proposed the possibility of adding a new drug to her treatment regimen. He was concerned that they were losing ground with her arthritis, even though Earlene was on a pretty potent treatment program. He didn't like the continued evidence of disease activity, particularly in the joints. Although the rash and fever hadn't returned, it now appeared that she had a condition resembling chronic rheumatoid arthritis. That is one of three possible outcomes of adult Still's disease, the other two being remission or continued episodes of fever, rash, and arthritis.

If the arthritis continued to smolder, Earlene would almost certainly suffer joint damage, which would likely result in disability. To avoid this, the doctor revisited the idea of TNF-alpha inhibitors.

TNF-alpha inhibitors. These biological anti-inflammatory agents block inflammation directly by interfering with the action of TNF-alpha, a potent chemical produced by inflammatory cells. We now have three such agents, and other promising biological therapies are under investigation.

The doctor noted that although all three TNF inhibitors were effective, none had been in use long enough for doctors to have a clear idea what the long-term side effects might be. Nevertheless, he chose to start her on infliximab because it had been in use somewhat longer than the other two. The main disadvantage of infliximab as compared to etanercept and adalimumab is that infliximab has to be given intravenously, while etanercept and adalimumab can be injected under the skin by the patient, like a diabetic giving herself an insulin shot.

So, after making sure that Earlene's tuberculosis skin test was negative, her doctor started her on infliximab intravenous therapy, eventually lengthening the time between doses from two to six weeks. Although it took a few weeks, Earlene's response to treatment was excellent.

What to Expect

As noted above, Still's disease may follow one of three possible courses. It can continue a relapsing course, with episodes of active arthritis, fever, and rash separated by inactive periods of varying length during which you may not have to take any medications. Second, it may go into a complete and permanent remission with no need for treatment. Third, it may metamorphose into something that looks a lot like garden-variety rheumatoid arthritis, with chronic arthritis, but no fever or rash. If the latter course occurs, treatment is just like that for rheumatoid arthritis and is necessary to prevent joint destruction.

Will I be disabled?

Joint destruction and disability are likely only if the rheumatoid arthritis–like course ensues, and then only if treatment is delayed or the disease does not respond to aggressive treatment. This is the course that Earlene's disease took, but because she responded so well to treatment, she did not have any resultant disability.

Disease at a Glance: Adult Still's Disease

Who Gets It?

- Very rare
- Men and women
- May or may not be hereditary

Joint Involvement

- Many joints; episodic activity initially
- If chronic, joint destruction is common in both large and small joints; tends to occur in the same joints on both sides of body

Other Features and Complications

- Episodic fever and rash
- Koebner's phenomenon
- Sore throat

Lab Results

- Elevated acute-phase reactants (sedimentation rate and C-reactive protein)
- Negative blood test for rheumatoid factor

Treatment

- General
  - Adequate rest
  - Appropriate exercise
  - Education
- Medications
  - Aspirin or other NSAID
  - Systemic corticosteroid during acute episodes (usually prednisone)
  - Antimalarial drug, such as hydroxychloroquine
  - Methotrexate and/or other DMARD
  - TNF-alpha inhibitor or IL-1 inhibitor, such as etanercept
  - Local joint injections with corticosteroids
- Surgery if appropriate

Earlene's Outcome

At this writing, Earlene continues to do well. She and Fred are planning to get married, with Gladys to be the matron of honor. Oscar, the young medical student who made the initial diagnosis, struck up a friendship with Gladys and Fred and kept in touch with Earlene's progress.

Chapter 8

Systemic Lupus Erythematosus

Onset: A Sunburn to Remember

Phyllis was 24 years old and just starting her new job as an apprentice grave-digger for the Municipal Cemetery Association. Although she had a bachelor's degree in biology, she had been unable to find work that took advantage of her hard-won skills and also paid a living wage. She had joined the steelworkers union, which had a section for grave-diggers, and she was ready to go to work. She was a husky young woman who had done construction work during summer breaks from college, and she was looking forward to the outdoor work her new job required. Phyllis had learned to operate a backhoe on her construction job, and that experience was going to stand her in very good stead. The training in biology didn't look like it was going to be of much value to her, but you never could tell.

It was a hot, sunny August, and the first week Phyllis was basically occupied with learning her way around the cemetery and working with old Enoch, the senior grave-digger, who had been with Municipal for 38 years and kept talking about retiring. Then one day Enoch got sick—sunstroke, they said—and Phyllis was left to carry the load. That

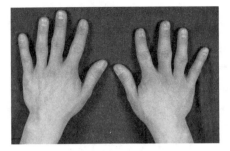

Figure 8-1: Hands of a patient with systemic lupus erythematosus and arthritis affecting many of the small joints of the fingers. This arthritis is usually not destructive, although it can rarely cause some deformity.

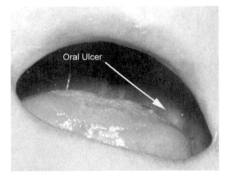

Oral Ulcer

Figure 8-2: Mouth ulcers, typically surrounded by a white base, are common in patients with active lupus. They may or may not be painful.

was okay with her because now she would get a chance to show her new employers what she was made of.

Because it was hot and nobody else was around, Phyllis shed her shirt and worked in her tank top. She heaved to it with a will and dug more graves in a shorter time than Municipal had ever seen. Her graves were very neat, perfectly rectangular, laid out accurately in the prescribed relationship with the adjacent graves, and exactly six feet deep, just the way the bosses wanted them. By the end of the day, Phyllis was extensively sunburned on her face and much of her upper body, but she felt good. She put her shirt back on and left for home, looking forward to a shower and a cool drink with her boyfriend, Harold.

Phyllis and Harold enjoyed a convivial evening, and when he went home about ten o'clock, she fell into bed and went to sleep immediately. The next morning, however, she was weak and achy and felt as if she were coming down with some sort of viral infection. Her hands and wrists were particularly painful, and when she examined them, they appeared to be moderately swollen. Phyllis looked in the mirror a few minutes later and saw a scaling rash on her face. When she ran a comb through her hair, more than the normal amount of hair stuck in the comb. Her mouth was sore, and in the mirror she could see what looked like shallow sores inside her cheek and on the roof of her mouth, both of which were white.

Phyllis knew something was wrong. She decided to take her temperature, noting that she was feeling alternately hot and cold. The thermometer read 103 degrees. Phyllis got herself dressed, hauled herself somewhat painfully into her ancient Yugo, and headed for the internist's office.

Phyllis's Assessment

When Phyllis arrived, she immediately had to urinate and, unusually for her, barely made it to the ladies' room in time. She discharged what seemed to her to be a very large amount of foamy urine. In the process, she noticed that her legs were a bit swollen.

As she returned to the waiting room, she heard the receptionist call her name, and she was quickly ushered into an examining room. The nurse took her temperature and blood pressure and instructed her to disrobe and put on a gown. She also asked Phyllis for a urine sample. Considering how recently Phyllis had emptied her bladder, she was surprised at how much more urine she was able to produce.

The doctor entered the room moments later and asked Phyllis to describe her problem. After she told him, he inquired about her previous health status, which had always been excellent, and that of her parents and two brothers. Also excellent. He then examined her carefully, taking her blood pressure again, looking closely at her rash, the sores in her mouth, her swollen finger joints, and the swelling in her legs, which was severe enough that he could make deep impressions in her flesh with his fingers.

"Phyllis, this might seem like a silly question, but when you get cold, do you notice any color changes in your hands?" he asked.

Surprised, she replied, "My hands have always been sensitive to the cold. When I get cold, my fingers turn dead white, then blue, and as I warm them up, they get very red and feel like they are on fire. How did you know that?"

Phyllis had just given a textbook description of a condition called Raynaud's phenomenon. What's more, her temperature had gone up to 103.5, and her blood pressure was elevated to 160 over

100, moderately higher than the norm for her age, which is about 115 over 74. Also, her urine sample contained a large amount of protein along with a little blood.

All of this led the doctor to believe that Phyllis might have a condition called systemic lupus erythematosus (SLE) and that it might be affecting her kidneys. This is a serious diagnosis, so he immediately admitted Phyllis to the hospital, where a rheumatologist could see her, confirm the diagnosis, and put her on a treatment program right away.

At that point, the doctor wrote orders for some blood and urine tests and X-rays and sent Phyllis, along with the faithful Harold, over to the hospital to arrange for her admission and the initial testing. They spent the rest of the day getting Phyllis settled into her room, with a parade of people—staff physicians, doctors-in-training, nurses, technicians, and so on—passing through, asking questions, prodding and poking her, and obtaining samples of blood and urine.

Later, Phyllis's internist introduced her and Harold to the rheumatologist. The new doctor examined her, talked with them about her condition, outlined a plan for the next few days, and discussed starting her on treatment. After briefly reviewing the lab results that were available by then, the rheumatologist told Phyllis that many of the most important results would be forthcoming over the next couple of days, but he was pleased to report that her kidney function appeared to be good. Her white blood count was low (another diagnostic criterion for SLE), but her red cell count was normal. The antinuclear antibody test, which measures antibody directed at components of the cell nucleus, was strongly positive (yet another criterion), but the more specific autoantibody test results were not yet available.

All about Systemic Lupus Erythematosus

Systemic lupus erythematosus (SLE or lupus for short) is a chronic disease of the immune system. The normal role of the immune system is to recognize large molecules—proteins, polysaccharides, lipids, and nucleic acids—and decide whether or not they belong in your body. When these large molecules interact with the immune system, they are called antigens and the result of exposure to "foreign" antigens is the production of proteins that bind to them, called antibodies. The decision as to whether or not the antigen in question belongs in the body depends on whether the immune system recognizes it as native, or "self" (it belongs there), or foreign, or "not self" (doesn't belong there).

If the antigen is foreign, the immune system attacks it by producing large amounts of antibodies against it. Antibodies are a part of the normal protection system that gets rid of harmful bacteria and viruses that may get into the circulation. In lupus and other autoimmune diseases, the ability of the immune system to make this distinction is impaired. People affected with lupus make large amounts of autoantibodies that react against their own molecules, whether they are in cells, on cells, or floating freely in the circulation. Many of these autoantibodies are harmful and cause the various disease manifestations that we refer to as lupus.

Depending, at least in part, on the array of autoantibodies produced, the disease has somewhat different characteristics in different people. In SLE, some of these autoantibodies react with components of cell nuclei, which are released into the circulation when cells come to the end of their lifespan and undergo destruction. The most characteristic autoantibodies found in people with SLE are those against DNA, the building blocks of genes, but there are other autoantibodies against cell components as well (for example, anti-Sm, anti-Ro/SSA, anti-La/SSB, and others). In the bloodstream, these autoantibodies combine with their antigens and form immune complexes that can move through the circulation and be deposited in various parts of the body, where they cause inflammation.

A common location for this deposition of immune complexes is the filtration membranes of the kidneys. When this happens, the filtration process is disrupted. This is one of the important mechanisms by which waste products are removed from the body.

Proteins in the blood, which are normally too large to infiltrate the kidney membranes, can now pass through. That causes elevated protein levels in the urine. Such immune complexes can deposit themselves elsewhere as well: for instance, in the skin, causing a rash; in the joint membranes, causing arthritis; and in other organs of the body, causing a variety of problems.

What causes systemic lupus erythematosus?

The cause of SLE is unknown. Genetics appear to play a role, and there is a tendency for SLE to occur in families where other members have lupus and other autoimmune diseases. But the genetics of SLE are not simple and straightforward. Multiple genes are probably involved, and environmental factors, for example viruses or drugs, may play a role as well.

SLE is not known to be contagious, and we think that it isn't. But there have been some intriguing observations that raise questions about this assumption. For instance, family dogs in households where someone has SLE have been reported to have laboratory findings suggestive of SLE. Laboratory personnel who handle blood from people with SLE have a higher than expected prevalence of positive tests for antinuclear antibodies. Many viral infections cause temporary elevations of antinuclear antibody levels in people who don't have SLE.

Some have suggested that SLE could be caused by a virus, but this has not been proven. With the interest in retroviruses generated by the AIDS epidemic, the possibility of a hard-to-detect virus that disappears into the genetic apparatus of infected cells has certainly received some attention, and the detection of antibody activity that seemed to be directed against the HTLV-I retrovirus in patients with lupus caused a lot of excitement a few years ago. But as of now, all we really have on this point are a number of tantalizing clues and no definitive proof of anything.

What are the symptoms of systemic lupus erythematosus?

There are 11 criteria that we use to diagnose SLE. These were defined and validated by the American College of Rheumatology back in the 1980s, and they are accepted around the world. If you have an illness in which any four of these are present, the diagnosis is very likely to be SLE (Phyllis had four). The degree of certainty increases with more than four criteria.

ACR (American College of Rheumatology) Criteria for the Diagnosis of Systemic Lupus Erythematosus

- Rash on the cheeks (butterfly rash)
- Discoid rash (raised, round, red patches)
- Sun sensitivity (photosensitivity)
- Sores on the mouth or nose
- Nondeforming arthritis
- Pleurisy (inflammation of the membrane surrounding the lungs) or pericarditis (inflammation of the membrane surrounding the heart)
- Kidney disorder: protein (proteinuria) or cellular casts in the urine (aggregations of red blood cells)
- Convulsions or psychosis
- Low blood level of white cells or platelets, or hemolytic anemia (low red cell count due to destruction of red cells caused by antibodies)
- Immunologic disorder: positive LE (lupus erythematosus) cell test, positive anti-double-stranded DNA test, positive anti-Sm test, positive anticardiolipin, or false-positive syphilis test
- Positive ANA (antinuclear antibody) test

A first episode of SLE is often provoked by sun exposure, although certain other events can trigger it as well. So the first clue in Phyllis's case was the onset of disease after unusual sun exposure and sunburn. That is called photosensitivity, and it is one of the hallmarks of SLE. Also, Phyllis had arthritis affecting the small joints of her hands. Arthritis is a second criterion for SLE. This type of arthritis tends to be nondeforming—that is, unlikely to damage the joints permanently, as rheumatoid arthritis frequently does.

A third clue to Phyllis's diagnosis was the sores in her mouth. Oral ulcerations, painful or not, are a criterion for the diagnosis of SLE, as are elevated protein levels in the urine. This is called proteinuria, and it too is a hallmark of SLE. Phyllis's urine sample displayed such elevated levels.

In addition, the unusual hair loss (alopecia) that Phyllis noticed also suggests lupus, although it is not a formal criterion. Another suggestive symptom is Raynaud's phenomenon, which Phyllis described so well. Finally, there were her lab results: a low white blood count and a strongly positive antinuclear antibody test, both being criteria for diagnosis of SLE.

If you exhibit at least four of the ACR criteria for SLE, the likelihood of the diagnosis being SLE is greater than 90 percent.

What other tests do I need?

Most critical for Phyllis was an evaluation of her kidney function. Kidney damage is probably the biggest immediate threat with SLE. Other onerous complications include central nervous system symptoms and impaired blood coagulation, which brings about excessive bleeding and bruising.

In order to evaluate the severity of any kidney disease, your doctor will need to obtain a biopsy specimen from one of your kidneys. The biopsy will reveal whether or not all parts of the kidneys are involved (diffuse disease) as opposed to spotty involvement (focal disease). Your doctor will also get a look at the nature of the inflammation in the filtration system—the glomeruli—of the kidneys, and see if it's aggressively inflammatory and rapidly progressive (proliferative) as opposed to mildly inflammatory and slowly progressive (membranous) or something in between (membranoproliferative). Using a modern electron microscope, we can even see the immune complex deposits and determine where they're located with respect to the filtering membrane; this gives us additional information about the disease's aggressiveness.

Finally, a kidney biopsy can help your doctor determine to what degree the process is reversible. Once scarring occurs from unchecked inflammation, it is no longer reversible. This is called glomerulosclerosis. If scarring is widespread, risky treatment has no purpose, and the next step may be to consider dialysis and kidney transplantation. Dialysis is the use of an artificial kidney machine at regular intervals (usually about three times weekly) to filter waste products from the blood, accumulated because of poor kidney function. Kidney transplantation is the process of implanting a healthy kidney, from either a living donor (usually a relative) or a recently deceased donor who was in good health up until the time of death.

How is a kidney biopsy obtained? There are two techniques for carrying out a kidney biopsy. The least invasive way is to place a biopsy needle in the kidney through the skin of the upper back under local anesthesia and withdraw a tissue sample. This often works out very well, and pain associated with this approach tends to be minimal, but several things can go wrong. First, because the procedure is normally done without X-ray guidance, we can miss the kidney entirely and get no tissue, or we can get an inadequate sample that does not contain enough kidney filtration units for analysis. Second, we can't always tell immediately if the kidney, which has many blood vessels, is bleeding after the biopsy specimen is obtained. This can lead to internal bleeding that may not be recognized right away. Open surgery may be necessary to correct either of these problems if they occur.

The second approach—generally preferred as safer—is to harvest the tissue specimen by way of open surgery, where we can see what we are getting, be sure to obtain a satisfactory sample, and make certain that there's no bleeding afterward. The disadvantages of an open biopsy are that it requires general anesthesia and the postoperative pain can be significant. The surgical incision also takes longer to heal than a needle puncture, and it leaves a visible scar.

Phyllis's doctor explained to her that, either way, if all went well, it would take a few days before the results were in and he could determine the course of treatment. He recommended that in the meantime she be started on a medication to keep things in check.

Is SLE genetic?

There does appear to be a hereditary component in lupus, which tends to run in families. There is a 10 percent likelihood that a family member of a lupus patient will also have it, and a 69 percent likelihood that an identical twin will also have it. Some hereditary antigens on white cells (HLA antigens A1, B8, DR2, DR3, and DQ1) are more common in SLE than in the population at large. But it is unlikely that genetics tells the whole story. It seems that some people inherit the susceptibility to SLE, but in reality, anyone can get it.

SLE and pregnancy

There are three basic issues to consider:

- Will you be able to carry a pregnancy through to term with a healthy baby?
- Would a pregnancy be safe for you?
- What treatment will you need for lupus, and what is its possible effect on the baby?

SLE may have implications for all of these issues.

Carrying a pregnancy to term with a healthy baby SLE per se generally doesn't affect a person's fertility, so getting pregnant would probably be no problem. But two conditions can occur in some women with lupus that may make it difficult to carry a pregnancy to completion. The more common of these is the presence of autoantibodies that adversely affect coagulation. Women with high levels of such antibodies often have miscarriages and have great difficulty carrying pregnancies to term, probably because once bleeding starts, the coagulation system can't stop it or because coagulation within the blood vessels, caused by antibodies, interrupts the circulation to the placenta.

One of the tests Phyllis underwent is an assay for anticardiolipin antibodies in the blood. Cardiolipin is a lipoprotein antigen similar to that used in the Venereal Disease Research Laboratory (VDRL) test for syphilis; many people with SLE and certain other diseases possess antibodies that react with this antigen. If high levels of such antibodies are present, one result may be a tendency to miscarry. They have other implications as well, increasing the risk of stroke, bleeding into the lungs, and many additional effects of disordered coagulation.

The second condition is the presence of a particular antinuclear antibody called anti-SSA/Ro. This antibody sometimes cross-reacts with fetal heart tissue, and it can cause an abnormal heart rhythm in the baby that may not be compatible with life.

The safety of a pregnancy for a mother with lupus All of us who take care of patients with this disease consider pregnancy to be highly risky for mothers with SLE because of the observed frequency of flare-ups during or immediately after pregnancy, even after long periods of relative lupus inactivity. That doesn't mean a person couldn't try it, but there's a significant risk. It's certainly not advisable to become pregnant while the disease is active; that's asking for trouble.

The effect that treatment might have on the developing fetus Many lupus treatments have the potential of interfering with normal fetal development. This is particularly true of chemotherapy drugs used for suppressing the immune system in severe cases. The risk of fetal death in this setting is considerable, but there's also a risk of producing an abnormal fetus that survives. But many lupus patients who have responded to treatment and no longer show evidence of active disease, can have normal pregnancies and healthy children. So pregnancy is not out of the question.

Does SLE predispose me to other diseases?

People with SLE occasionally develop Sjögren's syndrome (see chapter 2), which is characterized by dryness of the mouth and eyes as well as other normally moist surfaces. This condition carries an increased risk of developing a malignancy. Fortunately, it's pretty unusual.

Can SLE be prevented?

There is no known way to prevent systemic lupus erythematosus.

Can diet help?

Unfortunately, no autoimmune disease can be improved significantly by dietary means.

Should I exercise if I have SLE?

Systemic lupus erythematosus requires no specific exercise other than the normal physical activities that everyone should do for cardiovascular fitness. If the arthritic component of lupus is active, it is a good rule of thumb not to repeat any exercise that produces joint pain lasting more than two hours.

How common is SLE?

Although the statistics for systemic lupus erythematosus are not considered completely reliable, the best ones available are from a survey recently published by the American College of Rheumatology. It reports that 161,000 to 322,000 Americans have SLE. For unknown reasons, lupus mostly affects young women. It is much less common for men or older people to develop SLE, but it certainly can occur.

Treating Systemic Lupus Erythematosus

Can SLE be cured?

As with many autoimmune diseases, we do not currently have a cure for SLE. However, most people with the disease respond to treatment and live long, productive lives. Some even go into prolonged or permanent remissions, get completely off medications, live to a ripe old age, and die of something else. But some people do die of SLE or its complications, including side effects of treatment.

What factors are considered when choosing a treatment plan?

The acuteness of the disease process and the organ systems involved are the most important factors. SLE is complex, and the medicines used to treat both the underlying disease and its complications—such as hypertension, convulsive seizures, and antiphospholipid syndrome (described shortly), to name a few—are potent and have many side effects.

In choosing a treatment plan, it is important to avoid potentially toxic combinations of medicines as well as medicines that are rendered highly toxic by the patient's condition. An example of the latter would be the use of cyclophosphamide—a powerful immunosuppressive drug often used in SLE with active kidney disease—in a person with impaired kidney function. If your kidneys don't work properly, you can't excrete the drug normally, leading to higher than expected levels of the drug in the bloodstream.

As you will see, this was one of the medications used to treat Phyllis. The blood tests and any biopsy results are key to determining an appropriate course of treatment for SLE.

Phyllis's Treatment

Phyllis's doctor determined that there would be at least two phases to her treatment: what they did immediately and what they did when all the information came back from the laboratory.

Medication

The doctor started Phyllis on a moderately high dose of prednisone, 60 milligrams daily. It's not adequate to treat severe SLE, and it's overkill for mild disease. But it's a reasonable compromise, and it would buy them a little time to get the information necessary to develop a more tailored program. Since Phyllis would be taking the drug at that dosage for only about a week, the doctor told her not to worry about side effects. However, over the long haul, prednisone can have significant adverse effects in addition to the beneficial ones.

The test results

Phyllis's blood coagulation tests were normal, and her health was good other than the recent symptoms of SLE. Her anticardiolipin levels were not elevated. Her anti-DNA level, on the other hand, was very high, which is consistent with active SLE, and her complement levels were low. Complement is a system of proteins in the blood, similar to the coagulation system, which is activated by inflammatory antigen-antibody complexes. Complement is consumed in the process of generating inflammation; therefore in SLE, a low complement level usually means that the disease is active.

Phyllis recovered uneventfully from the kidney biopsy, but she did experience some soreness that continued for several days, requiring pain medication. The day after the procedure, the rheumatologist came into her hospital room and said that he had looked at the biopsy and discussed it with the pathologist. Although there were a few more studies to perform on the specimens, mainly electron microscopy, he had a preliminary report.

The good news was that, as he'd expected, there was no scarring in the kidney, and he felt confident that aggressive treatment would preserve most of Phyllis's kidney function. The bad news was that the inflammation from lupus was diffuse, involving all the glomeruli that could be seen in the specimen. The nature of the inflammation was proliferative, meaning that the process was acute and needed treatment right away. This condition is called diffuse proliferative glomerulonephritis. If left untreated, it can destroy kidney function.

What is the treatment of SLE with diffuse proliferative glomerulonephritis?

The moderately high dose of prednisone produced very positive results for Phyllis. All her aches and pains were gone, except for the soreness relating to the biopsy. Even her mouth was healing. Unfortunately, she couldn't continue to take 60 milligrams of prednisone a day indefinitely because of side effects. The doctor prescribed a medication called cyclophosphamide, administered intravenously at monthly intervals. Phyllis received her first dose that day while still in the hospital. Assuming that she tolerated the medication without difficulty, she would be discharged from the hospital the next day. The doctor also directed Phyllis to return for monthly follow-up visits.

What are the side effects of these treatments?

Prednisone As mentioned earlier, prednisone has many side effects. The most noticeable one is a tendency to gain weight. Prednisone strongly stimulates the appetite, and almost everybody who takes it in anything more than the smallest dosage gains weight. The distribution of the newly acquired body fat is different from normal obesity, settling in the trunk and the face, while the arms and legs remain thin. The appearance of someone on prednisone is characteristic, and people familiar with the drug's effects will be able to tell that you are taking it. Fortunately, this whole process is reversible upon stopping the drug, although it takes some time off prednisone for things to return to normal.

Prednisone reduces a person's resistance to infection, and people taking it in doses higher than 20 milligrams daily often get infections, which may be severe. These infections respond normally to antibiotics, but it is important to recognize them early and get treatment started in a timely manner. Unfortunately, prednisone also masks some of the signs of infection that you would normally be watching for—fever, for example—so this is not as easy as it sounds.

Prednisone frequently causes osteoporosis, which is reduced bone strength due to low calcium content. This makes bones soft and increases the likelihood of fractures. We can somewhat reduce this effect by having you take supplemental calcium and vitamin D, but your bone density will need close monitoring.

Finally, prednisone can cause hypertension, diabetes, acne, thinning and bruising of the skin, and other problems.

Cyclophosphamide Cyclophosphamide is a chemotherapy drug belonging to the class referred to as alkylating agents. It is chemically similar to nitrogen mustard, so called because of its chemical resemblance to the mustard gas used in World War I. Cyclophosphamide works by binding to DNA in rapidly dividing cells and killing them. In active SLE, the most rapidly dividing cells are the immune cells producing autoantibodies that cause the disease, as well as the inflammatory cells themselves. The goal of using this drug is to wipe out the populations of antibody-producing cells without doing permanent harm to the rest of the immune system or other cells of the body. Most of cyclophosphamide's side effects result from its tendency to attack other dividing cells at the same time it is doing what we want it to do.

Because cyclophosphamide is excreted in the urine, the urinary bladder is exposed to the medication until it empties. The drug can have two very bad effects on the bladder:

- Cyclophosphamide can irritate the bladder wall and cause hemorrhaging. This can be very severe, and a person can actually bleed to death. So if you are taking this drug and see any sign of blood in your urine, that is a potential emergency, and you should call your doctor immediately.

- Irritation of the bladder wall can, over time, lead to bladder cancer. This can be treated, but therapy generally calls for removal of the urinary bladder. If you were to take cyclophosphamide by mouth, your bladder would be exposed to it all the time you're taking the drug. By giving it in monthly intravenous doses, however, your doctor can minimize the exposure of the bladder to the drug. Furthermore, a chemoprotective drug called mesna is often administered along with the cyclophosphamide to protect the bladder wall. You must be vigilant about both of these adverse effects, so that if they occur, they can be treated as early as possible. Although bladder cancer is the most frequent type of malignancy caused by cyclophosphamide, it can also cause other forms, especially lymphoma and leukemia, and your doctor will want to watch for these as well.

- Cyclophosphamide, like many forms of chemotherapy, also can induce nausea and vomiting. To prevent this, each administration of cyclophosphamide and mesna is typically accompanied by a dose of ondansetron, a strong antinausea medication. This usually completely prevents nausea and vomiting.

- Cyclophosphamide is also prone to cause hair loss. With the dosage of cyclophosphamide used in treating SLE, we sometimes see it, but certainly not always. This hair loss, though it can lead to total baldness, is completely reversible: when the drug is stopped after the course of treatment is finished, the hair grows back normally. Some people like to have a wig on hand just in case, but I would recommend waiting to spend money on a wig, because in most people the hair loss is not severe enough to be noticeable.

- Cyclophosphamide can also suppress the bone marrow, where blood cells are manufactured. Suppression of the bone marrow can result in anemia, or a low red-cell count; leukopenia, or a low white-cell count; and thrombocytopenia, or a low platelet count. Red cells carry oxygen throughout the circulation to the whole body, and severe anemia can deprive body organs of enough oxygen for normal function. The most common symptoms of anemia are tiredness, lack of energy, and easy fatigability. White cells are important in the body's defense against infection, and leukopenia makes a person more susceptible to germs. Platelets are essential to normal blood coagulation, and severe thrombocytopenia can lead to prolonged bleeding and poor clot formation.

- Cyclophosphamide can also cause sterility by directly damaging the ovaries.

Azathioprine Phyllis's doctor informed her that once the course of cyclophosphamide was completed (during which they would gradually reduce the dose of prednisone), he wanted to start her on oral azathioprine. This drug also suppresses the immune system but not as strongly as cyclophosphamide. Recent studies have shown that remissions induced by cyclophosphamide are maintained more effectively by taking a moderate dosage of azathioprine afterward. But azathioprine also has side effects:

- Azathioprine can suppress the bone marrow in much the same manner as cyclophosphamide, leading to anemia, leukopenia, and thrombocytopenia.

- Azathioprine can also exert toxic effects on the liver. Your doctor will need to watch for signs of liver dysfunction by ordering various sensitive blood tests at regular intervals while you take this medication.

What benefit can I expect from treatment?

The treatment plan outlined for Phyllis is, in my opinion, the best form of therapy that we currently have for lupus with severe kidney disease. In such a situation, we are trying to do two things: keep you alive and preserve your kidneys. If we accomplish both goals, treatment will have been successful. But in addition, we usually induce a complete remission of the systemic disease, so the bothersome but not particularly dangerous symptoms you had at the beginning, including the arthritis, should be gone. We try to spare you from serious side effects, and we usually succeed.

Nevertheless, sometimes we cannot totally control the disease, and it recurs. If this happens, we simply repeat the course of medications. The risk of side effects is greater the second time around, but we still usually get by with it. If this happens repeatedly, however, you could lose kidney function over time, possibly resulting in the need for dialysis and kidney transplantation. That is certainly not the ideal outcome, but even patients who must undergo transplantation usually do very well, especially if the transplanted kidney comes from a living, related donor.

What other treatments are there for SLE?

Recently there has been interest in treating lupus by depleting a class of white blood cells called B lymphocytes. These are the cells responsible for antibody production. Since autoantibodies probably play a major role in producing many of the nasty features of lupus, this approach makes sense, and it was the basis of one of the early treatments for lupus called plasmapheresis. In this treatment, which may sound a bit drastic, blood plasma was removed from a vein in the patient's arm using a special machine available in blood banks, thus getting rid of antibodies thought to be causing problems. It was impractical because antibodies were replaced about as fast as they could be removed. However, we now have biological agents that can effectively remove B cells. They are normally used to treat certain forms of lymphatic cancer, but there is interest in testing their effectiveness in lupus. The agent with the most experience behind it is rituximab, but this is not mainstream therapy for lupus as yet.

What to Expect

Severe kidney disease is one of several serious forms that lupus can take. Although SLE can cause problems in almost any system of the body, there are two other major problems that could arise, and all SLE patients should be on the alert for them. Statistically, if they don't occur in the first couple of years, they become somewhat less likely ever to happen in a given person.

If SLE affects the central nervous system, it can cause very severe problems, the most dramatic of which are strokes, convulsive seizures, and psychoses.

- Strokes look just like the typical strokes that people can get with arteriosclerosis—hardening of the arteries—in which some neurological functions suddenly stop. One side of the body can become paralyzed, sometimes with loss of speech and some mental functions. This can lead to permanent disability, and, if vital centers of the brain, especially the brain stem, are affected, a person could die. The big difference between these strokes and the more common variety is that lupus-induced strokes tend to occur in younger people.

- Seizures can be total body convulsions (grand mal) or more limited (petit mal), in which the affected person may or may not recognize that something has happened. Either way, patients need to be treated with anticonvulsant medications.

- Psychosis can take the form of any mental disorder, or it can look more like an organic brain syndrome, in which the person loses short-term memory and becomes disoriented.

These neurological conditions vary in the degree to which they respond to standard SLE treatment, and in some cases there is disagreement about what the best treatment should be. Generally, they are treated with prednisone along with more specific therapy for the conditions they resemble: anticonvulsants for seizures or antipsychotic drugs for psychosis.

The other major condition occurs when antibodies form against components of the coagulation system. Although these antibodies are commonly referred to as lupus anticoagulants, they do not typically cause bleeding. Paradoxically, they cause trouble by activating the coagulation system so that clotting occurs spontaneously in the blood vessels, leading to blockage of the blood supply to the organs supplied by those blood vessels. This may be what happens in at least some forms of SLE-induced strokes, but it can occur in almost any organ.

This phenomenon appears to be responsible for spontaneous miscarriages in pregnant women with lupus. It is also associated with fatal hemorrhagic pneumonia in lupus. It can cause deep vein thrombophlebitis—that is, blood clots in the leg veins, which can break off and travel to the lungs (pulmonary embolus) and other organs. It can result in disseminated intravascular coagulation (DIC), with widespread gangrene caused by the blockage of blood circulation in many vessels, an often fatal condition. The modern name of this antibody-induced disorder of blood coagulation is antiphospholipid syndrome. The treatment for it is to recognize it before it causes problems by testing for antibodies against phospholipids—the typical one tested for is anticardiolipin—and treating aggressively with anticoagulants, usually warfarin. These antibodies often cause a false positive test for syphilis, which also uses the cardiolipin antigen.

Will I be disabled?

SLE, as an autoimmune disease, carries serious risks if untreated. However, the arthritis commonly associated with it is not destructive in the way that other arthritic conditions such as rheumatoid arthritis are. Your joints, though painful, will not be eroded or permanently damaged by the accompanying inflammation, but if left untreated, the joint pain may be significant.

Phyllis's Outcome

Phyllis tolerated the course of strong medicines the doctor prescribed for her. She gained about 30 pounds early on because of prednisone, but two years later she was on minimal doses of the prednisone and azathioprine, and was back to her original weight. She felt well. She and Harold had gotten married, but they decided to wait to start a family until Phyllis was off medication. That took another three years, during which she had no attacks of SLE, and her kidney function was normal.

Six years after the original attack, Phyllis and Harold decided that they had waited long enough. After consulting with her doctor, who gave his blessing, they took the necessary steps and Phyllis became pregnant. A high-risk obstetrician recommended by her rheumatologist monitored her pregnancy, and after nine uneventful months, she gave birth to a beautiful seven-pound daughter that

Disease at a Glance: Systemic Lupus Erythematosus

Who Gets It?
- Women 17 to 35 years old, predominantly
- More frequent and more severe in African-Americans
- Moderate heredity component
- 161,000 to 322,000 Americans affected

Joint involvement
- Small joints of hands and wrists affected most frequently
- Nondestructive arthritis
- Frequent avascular/aseptic necrosis (see glossary) of hips, knees, shoulders, especially with high-dose corticosteroid treatment
- Joints rarely the main problem (see Other Features and Complications)

Other Features and Complications
- Glomerulonephritis/kidney failure
- Convulsions or psychosis
- Pleurisy/pericarditis
- Antiphospholipid syndrome
  - Stroke
  - Multiple miscarriages
  - Hemorrhagic pneumonitis (bleeding into the lungs)
- Skin rash (malar distribution over the cheeks—called butterfly rash)
- Photosensitivity
- Hair loss
- Mouth sores

Lab Results
- Anemia, low white-cell count, low platelet count
- Antinuclear antibody (ANA)

(continued)

- Antibodies against DNA, other nuclear antigens
- False-positive syphilis test (due to antiphospholipid antibodies)
- Protein and red-cell casts (red cell aggregates) in the urine
- Low complement levels
- Elevated acute-phase reactants (such as sedimentation rate)

Treatment
- General
  — Adequate rest
  — Appropriate exercise
  — Education
  — Medications for arthritis and skin features
- Medications for arthritis and skin features
  — Aspirin or other NSAID
  — Antimalarial drug, such as hydroxychloroquine
- Medications for kidney and/or central nervous system features
  — Systemic corticosteroids, such as prednisone
  — Systemic immunosuppressive drugs, such as cyclophosphamide
- Other treatments as indicated for less common features

she and Harold named Hyacinth. Both the baby and the mother did fine. Phyllis continued to see her doctor at six-month intervals, and she and her family are doing well to this day.

Not everyone is so fortunate, as the obstetrician told Phyllis and Harold. By delaying pregnancy for so long after all signs of active lupus had abated, they had minimized but not eliminated the risk of a lupus flare. Even after many years of apparent quiescence, lupus can reactivate and be very difficult to control. But Phyllis, Harold, and Hyacinth (who is now in college) got through it unscathed, and that is what counts.

Chapter 9

Infectious Arthritis

Onset: What's a Joint Like This Doing in a Nice Girl Like You?

Frieda had just turned 64, and she was looking forward to retiring the following year. After more than 40 years of working as a maid and cleaning lady in the county hospital, she was about worn out. But she had a lot to be thankful for.

She had come to America from her childhood home in western Poland as a teenage orphan, speaking only German and Polish, and with little education, minimal cash, and no prospects. Through the church, she made some friends who spoke Polish and German, learned some English, and found work in the hospital.

She eventually met Jakob, a nice young steelworker only a couple of years older than she was. He courted her, and they married after a few months. Over the next five years, they had four children: two girls (Hannah and Hedwig) and two boys (Heinrich and Hermann).

Then, tragically, just after their tenth anniversary, when everything seemed to be going well, Jakob was killed in a freak accident at the plant. Although he had only a small insurance policy, the company had a fairly liberal attitude about its obligations to families of employees injured or killed on the job, and it agreed to provide a stipend to Frieda until her children were through school. This, together with her small salary from the hospital, enabled her to support the family. Eventually, all the children grew up, finished their educations, got jobs, got married, and moved to other cities, where there was greater opportunity for white-collar employment.

Frieda continued working without complaint and putting away her money. One day, shortly after her 64th birthday, she noticed that her right knee was a little stiff and sore, and it looked mildly swollen.

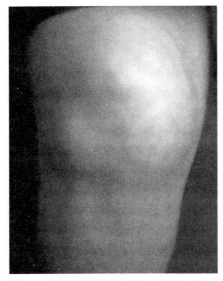

Figure 9-1: Swelling of a single knee (monoarthritis) is typical of infectious arthritis, although it may also be seen in several other conditions. In tuberculous arthritis, the inflammation is generally not as intense as in arthritis caused by pus-forming bacteria, like staph and strep.

She assumed that she had twisted it while carrying her scrub bucket up three flights of stairs, as she did every day. But the swelling didn't go down, and it seemed to get a little worse as the weeks wore on. Frieda was dependent on a reasonable degree of physical well-being in order to maintain her livelihood. Anything that might limit her capacity to work was a significant threat, so she decided not to put off consulting a physician any longer. She knew some of the doctors in the rheumatology department at the hospital where she worked. She liked them all, but she sought out a woman doctor who was fluent in German.

Frieda's Assessment

The doctor asked Frieda many questions about her general health and medical history, as well as any history of operations or injuries. Frieda had no chills, fever, weight loss, or any other symptoms suggesting chronic illness. She had experienced some sweating at night and hot flashes since she'd entered menopause some 15 years earlier. The doctor inquired in detail about Frieda's family medical history, but details were sketchy on this issue. Frieda couldn't remember much about her parents' health, and she had no brothers or sisters. She reported that her four children were all healthy and that her pregnancies had been uneventful.

Following this, the doctor examined Frieda carefully, paying particular attention to her skin; listening to her lungs through the stethoscope; feeling for enlarged lymph nodes, liver, and spleen; checking all her joints; and manipulating the right knee. The examination was pretty much normal except for the obvious swelling in the right knee, which was also mildly tender and warmer to the touch than the left knee.

The doctor determined that Frieda was suffering from a condition in the right knee that rheumatologists refer to as monoarticular arthritis. Most forms of arthritis affect several or many joints, but monoarticular arthritis involves only one. While several conditions can lead to monoarticular arthritis, the most likely causes are an infection in the joint or crystal-induced arthritis such as gout or pseudogout. Frieda's medical history and lack of family knowledge didn't provide many useful leads, so the doctor suggested a joint fluid aspiration. The most straightforward approach to making the correct diagnosis in a situation like Frieda's is to remove some fluid from the joint cavity through a needle, then examine it under the microscope and analyze it for cell content, protein content, and bacteria in the laboratory. The doctor removed several syringes full of cloudy yellow synovial (joint) fluid, placing small amounts into several sterile containers that would be used for culture and analysis.

Frieda was also sent for some blood tests and X-rays. Since her knee was not acutely painful, the doctor felt confident waiting for the test results before starting any treatment, provided that she didn't see any crystals in the joint fluid.

The doctor considered placing a tuberculosis skin test on Frieda's arm, but she knew that, beginning in the 1920s, vaccination with a TB-like bacterium called BCG (Bacillus Calmette-Guérin) was widely used in many countries to build immunity against tuberculosis. It is variably effective in preventing the disease (from 0 to 76 percent in several studies), but it almost always causes the tuberculosis skin test to convert to positive (and Frieda revealed that this was the case with her), thus rendering the usual skin test ineffective for diagnosing tuberculosis. In the United States, the Centers for Disease Control and Prevention (CDC) does not recommend routine use of BCG immunization because of its variable effectiveness in preventing tuberculosis and the relatively low risk of contracting this disease in this country. For Frieda, however, the decision had already been made.

The microscopic examination of the joint fluid did not reveal any crystals, but many inflammatory cells were present. This was not surprising, since the knee had the swelling and warmth suggestive of a chronic inflammatory process.

Frieda went off to the lab for blood testing and to the X-ray department for knee and chest X-rays, then she went back to work.

A week later, Frieda reported to the doctor's office. She was shocked to hear that she had tuberculous arthritis of the knee. The tuberculosis bacterium grew out of her joint fluid in the laboratory cultures, and it was also visible in the joint fluid under the microscope with special staining, so the doctor had no doubts about the diagnosis.

The most up-to-date diagnosis and treatment recommendations for tuberculosis can be found on the CDC website at www.cdc. gov/ncidod/dq/panel_2007.htm.

Although we normally think of tuberculosis as a disease of the lungs, the germ that causes tuberculosis—*Mycobacterium tuberculosis*—can sometimes infect other tissues. The lungs are the most commonly affected organs because the usual way this germ gets into the body is by being inhaled. But in Frieda's case, the bug settled in the right knee, and, luckily, that appeared to be the only site where it was now growing.

Because of the public health implications of tuberculosis, Frieda's doctor had to report the case to the health department, and she explained to Frieda that the health department would be participating in her treatment.

All about Infectious Arthritis

Tuberculous arthritis is one example of the broad category of infectious arthritis. It is like other cases of infectious arthritis in that the inflamed joint is directly infected with the microorganism responsible for the infection; in this case, *Mycobacterium tuberculosis*. Without treatment, infectious arthritis—whether low grade and subacute like tuberculosis or high grade and acute like staphylococcus or streptococcus—is extremely destructive and would ultimately destroy the joint. Tuberculous arthritis is unlike most other cases of infectious arthritis, which tend to be much more dramatic in onset, hotly inflamed, markedly swollen, and extremely painful, as well as destructive over a much shorter period of time. Despite the more chronic nature of tuberculous arthritis, the principles of diagnosis and treatment are the same, so it is a good example of infectious arthritis.

Although Frieda had received TB vaccinations as a child and had not been around anyone known to have tuberculosis for many years, she did work in the county hospital, which served the inner city. Many of the patients suffered from deficient immune systems due to AIDS and other conditions, which heightens their susceptibility to tuberculosis, and they can pass it on to others, mainly by coughing. If you go into many patients' rooms each day, as Frieda did, it is quite easy to become infected with something—after all, she was repeatedly exposed to any number of illnesses, most likely including tuberculosis.

Also, although tuberculosis is not as common in the United States as in many other countries, its frequency is significant here. That is a matter of concern to public health officials, especially since many of these cases, unlike in the past, are resistant to the usual forms of treatment.

Finally, Frieda had BCG vaccination against TB as a child. Unfortunately, BCG vaccination is nowhere nearly as effective against TB as, say, smallpox vaccination is against smallpox or polio vaccination is against polio. Even when it is effective, the effectiveness tends to decline over time. Frieda received BCG at least a half century previously, and it clearly didn't prevent the infection that she now had. The main thing that BCG did for her was to exclude her from participation in the hospital's TB surveillance program, which relies on annual skin tests for all employees.

What causes infectious arthritis?

Infectious arthritis, whether caused by a bacterium as in Frieda's case, a fungus, or a virus is due to direct invasion of a joint by a microorganism that grows in the joint and produces destructive inflammation. In most infectious arthritis cases, the offending agent gains entrance to the joint via the circulatory system, but occasionally it gets there more directly via a penetrating wound.

What are the symptoms of infectious arthritis?

The signs of joint infection are the same as the signs of noninfectious inflammation: swelling, warmth, pain, and impaired function (stiffness, for example). This may be chronic or subacute, as in Frieda's case; or very acute, as in the case of infection with a pus-forming bacterium such as staphylococcus or streptococcus.

Generally, the only way to make a definitive diagnosis is by aspirating the joint and examining the fluid under the microscope with special stains and by culturing it.

Most people look for fever as the first sign of an infection, and in most cases they would be right to do so. Frieda didn't have a fever when she went to see the doctor, but infectious arthritis may cause episodic fevers, not necessarily a constant one. Also, people sometimes have fever that isn't apparent to them. Not all fevers are accompanied by chills and shaking. The most common symptom of fever in people with tuberculosis is night sweats (which Frieda may have confused with her postmenopausal night sweats), and these tend to occur at the time the fever is breaking—that is, when the temperature is returning to normal. But some fevers are asymptomatic, and the only way you can detect them is by taking your temperature. However, some people with localized tuberculosis or other hidden infections do not have fever at all.

As noted above, most other bacteria cause a more acute infection than the tuberculosis bacterium does. A joint infected with staph, strep or some other pus-producing infectious agent tends to be tightly swollen, extremely tender, and very warm to the touch. Such bacteria are all around us in our daily lives, but, fortunately, most people avoid infection. People infected with these agents tend to have high fevers that remain elevated until they are treated with antibiotics. They also often have bacteria circulating in the blood, and blood cultures can lead to growth of the bacteria in the laboratory. People with such infections may be acutely ill and show classical signs of sepsis (systemic bacterial infection), such as fever and rigors, up to and including shock if the blood pressure drops to subnormal levels. These infections tend to be rapidly destructive, and they must be treated as medical emergencies.

Infectious funguses can also occasionally get into the joints and cause a form of arthritis that resembles tuberculous arthritis. They tend to get into the body either by inhalation or through breaks in the skin. They can make their way to the joints through the bloodstream. They're inflammatory, but the inflammation is usually of a lower grade than that caused by the pus-producing bacteria; it's subacute like tuberculosis rather than acute like staph. Many of these agents are prevalent in the environment as well. Some, like *Histoplasma capsulatum*, the fungus that causes histoplasmosis, and *Coccidioides immitis*, the fungus that causes coccidioidomycosis, have characteristic geographic distributions. In the United States, histoplasmosis is commonest in the Tennessee, Ohio, and Mississippi valleys, while coccidioidomycosis is most frequent in the San Joaquin Valley. When they infect the joints, these funguses are identified by examination of joint fluid.

Can infectious arthritis affect multiple joints?

Fortunately for Frieda, her TB was not very likely to spread to other joints. Most joint infections involve only one joint. A few infectious agents, the most familiar being gonorrhea, can get into multiple joints, but that rarely happens in tuberculosis.

Nevertheless, some bacteria and viruses can cause arthritis that is not due to direct infection of the joints, but rather to a generalized reaction of the body against the infection, and this situation often leads to arthritis in many joints. If you test the joint fluid from affected joints in such patients, the responsible infectious agent cannot be found there. These forms of arthritis are not generally thought of or referred to as infectious, but instead are classified as "reactive" to a remote infection.

Rheumatic fever arthritis Rheumatic fever arthritis, the most familiar example of this type of arthritis, is caused by the body's immune reaction against the streptococcus bacterium, which usually infects the throat. Strep throat is not to be taken lightly because it can lead to heart valve abnormalities. The immune system mistakes the body's own tissues for the streptococcus and attacks them. This occurs because certain chemicals on the surface of the streptococcus mimic chemicals in the human body. This phenomenon is called molecular mimicry, and it is one of the mechanisms underlying autoimmunity. The arthritis of rheumatic fever is generally mild and fleeting, and does little or no harm to the joints.

Poncet's arthritis Tuberculosis may also cause an immunologically generated arthritis called Poncet's arthritis. Antonin Poncet, a French surgeon, described it in 1897. It rarely occurs in people with tuberculosis, affects multiple joints, and may look like rheumatoid arthritis. This arthritis tends not to be destructive. The test for rheumatoid factor may be positive in such patients. No tuberculosis bacteria are found in the joint fluid, and the joint fluid is sterile, just as in rheumatic fever. Perhaps because this condition is very rare and would be found primarily in places where tuberculosis is common, American and British physicians are not sure that it exists. Since rheumatoid arthritis is also relatively common, the co-occurrence of these two diseases—tuberculosis and rheumatoid arthritis—in the same person would be expected to occur occasionally, and I suppose this could be an explanation for what we call Poncet's arthritis.

Is infectious arthritis genetic?

Like any infection, this type of arthritis is contracted. It does not appear to arise from a genetic predisposition.

Is infectious arthritis contagious?

Although Frieda's doctor cautioned her that she would need to take time off from work until her knee responded to treatment, she reassured her that she would ultimately be able to perform her job. She did have live, infectious TB germs in her body. But considering their location in the right knee and the lack of evidence that they had spread anywhere else, and also given that Frieda was not coughing, the doctor considered it unlikely that she was contagious. Coughing is the main mode by which this disease spreads, and Frieda probably got it by being around someone with TB who was coughing. Effective treatment was the surest way of preventing Frieda's tuberculosis from reentering her bloodstream and becoming contagious. If it were to reenter the circulation and make its way back to the lungs, she might begin coughing and thus could spread her TB to others.

How did the infection get to my knee?

The main route from the lungs to the joints or any other organ is the bloodstream, and that's probably what happened in Frieda's case. The most common joints affected by TB are those of the spine—the joints between the bones of the spine are called intervertebral joints—the hips, and the knees. When TB goes to the intervertebral joints, it's called Pott's disease after Percivall Pott, an English barber-surgeon who described tuberculosis of the spine in the 18th century.

Some people get lung TB, which becomes inactive, or latent, and sits there for many years without causing any problems. We can sometimes see this latent TB on a chest X-ray, where it appears as a calcified lesion called a Ghon focus, after Austrian pathologist Anton Ghon, who described it in 1912. Usually, this type of lesion doesn't progress, but occasionally, for unknown reasons, it activates and causes disease in the lungs or elsewhere. However, Frieda's chest X-ray showed no evidence of a Ghon focus or any other abnormality suggesting tuberculosis, so her doctor concluded that the initial infection had occurred fairly recently.

Does infectious arthritis predispose me to other diseases?

Infectious arthritis can damage the joint, which can lead to the development of osteoarthritis (see chapter 3) later, even after the infection is cured by antibiotics.

Can infectious arthritis be prevented?

Infectious agents can be inadvertently introduced into a joint during a joint aspiration for some other purpose or during joint surgery. That is why it is important that your physician use strict sterile technique when performing a joint aspiration.

Can diet help?

Diet has no known role in prevention or treatment of infectious arthritis.

Should I exercise if I have infectious arthritis?

Range-of-motion exercises are important during the recovery phase from infectious arthritis. Exercise would be excruciatingly painful in an untreated, acutely infected joint.

How common is infectious arthritis?

Reliable statistics are not available for the frequency of infectious arthritis.

Treating Infectious Arthritis

The principles of treating infectious arthritis are the same regardless of the type of infection. The goals are always to cure the infection and minimize or prevent damage to the infected joint. That means the sooner you get an accurate diagnosis and start treatment, the better off you are.

The tools of treatment are (1) protecting the infected joint by draining the inflammatory fluid as often as necessary and (2) getting rid of the infection by administering the proper antibiotics at the full dosage, by the most efficient route—by mouth, through a vein (intravenously, or IV), or by injection into muscle—and for the appropriate length of time. In many infections, although not in tuberculosis, the antibiotics must be given intravenously. This generally starts in the hospital, although once the acute phase of the infection is controlled and we are certain that the infection is responding to treatment, you may be able to have the antibiotics infused at home by a home health nurse.

Can infectious arthritis be cured?

The answer is yes, but in any case of infectious arthritis, use of the proper antibiotic for the appropriate length of time is essential in order to obtain a cure. Identification of the infecting organism through culturing fluid from the infected joint is absolutely critical, and testing of the organism in the laboratory for sensitivity to antibiotics is helpful for choosing the appropriate agent for treatment. Making sure that the antibiotic can get to the infection in the effective concentration is aided by repeatedly draining excess fluid from the infected joint until it ceases to accumulate.

As with other forms of infectious arthritis, tuberculosis in the knee can usually be cured using a combination of joint drainage and antibiotics specific for tuberculosis. The drug treatments we now have for tuberculosis are very effective and remarkably safe. But if the infection has caused any damage to the joint, the antituberculous treatment will not cure that. Any residual joint damage will need to be treated the way we treat osteoarthritis.

As in other infectious diseases, the medical treatment for tuberculosis has changed over time, and it's almost certain to continue to change as new antibiotics are developed and as the tuberculosis bacterium continues to evolve new drug-resistant strains. In 2003 the CDC, along with the American Thoracic Society and the Infectious Diseases Society of America, promulgated the current evidence-based guidelines for treatment, and these are what we use today to treat tuberculosis of the lungs, or pulmonary TB, and other organs, including the joints (extrapulmonary TB).

What factors are considered when choosing a treatment plan?

The culture and sensitivity data for the infectious agent is one piece of critical information. Another is the patient's drug allergy history. Allergy to many antibiotics is common, and your doctor's obtaining a comprehensive allergy history is one of the keys to successful treatment.

Frieda's Treatment

Medication

The doctor outlined a treatment plan beginning with what's called four-drug therapy, consisting of the antituberculous medications isoniazid, or INH; rifampin (RIF); pyrazinamide (PZA); and ethambutol (EMB). Fortunately, these drugs come in combination preparations, so Frieda only had to keep track of a few pills. For example, the brand-name drug Rifamate is a combination of INH and RIF, and Rifater is a combination of INH, RIF, and PZA. All four drugs were necessary at first because it wasn't yet clear if Frieda's particular TB germ was resistant to INH, as is frequently the case.

The doctor explained that the only way to determine how long to continue four-drug therapy is to test the bacterium that grows out of the joint fluid against INH and the other drugs. This is called sensitivity testing. The sensitivity test results from Frieda's knee-joint fluid cultures would help him decide which of the drugs she would need going forward. If her TB germ was sensitive to INH and RIF, then she could stop the EMB.

The physician also explained that during the initiation phase of treatment, Frieda would have to take her medications at the hospital daily for the next eight weeks so that the doctor could verify that she actually took them. This is called directly observed therapy, or DOT, and it is the standard method of treating tuberculosis and other diseases considered public health risks.

How long will treament last?

There are two phases to treating tuberculosis. The initiation phase, during which treatment is more intensive, lasts for eight weeks. In the continuation phase, which goes on for another twenty-six weeks, treatment is reduced. The total treatment takes about eight months, assuming that everything goes according to plan.

What are the side effects of treatment?

These drugs, like all drugs, have side effects. Although many side effects are possible, they are not particularly frequent with any of these drugs.

- INH can cause skin rash, stomach upset, side effects in the liver and the nervous system, and deficiency of the B vitamin pyridoxine.

- RIF can cause stomach upset, side effects in the liver and the kidneys, low platelet count, visual disturbances, menstrual irregularities, and swelling of the face and extremities.

- EMB can cause visual disturbances, skin rashes, itching, joint pain, gout, and side effects in the liver and the kidneys.

- PZA can cause stomach upset, joint pain, hives and itching, gout, and side effects in the liver.

Like most drugs, especially most antibiotics, all four antituberculosis drugs can cause allergic reactions in people who happen to be hypersensitive to them. If you are taking any of these drugs, you and your doctor will want to watch for these reactions. As long as you are monitored closely, these medications are pretty safe.

In more acute forms of infectious arthritis, where high doses of intravenous antibiotics may be given over several weeks, the normal bacterial content of the intestine can be altered, leading to diarrhea and possible infection with pathogenic agents like the bacterium *Clostridium difficile*, which may require some additional, different antibiotic treatment.

Frieda's Response to Treatment

"So, let's get started," suggested the doctor.

The doctor called in nurse Tyrone, and he assisted her in withdrawing fluid from Frieda's bad knee with a needle and syringe and gave Frieda the first doses of the four antituberculous drugs. She then asked Frieda to return the next day to see Tyrone to get her medications, and in one week to see her for recheck and further joint drainage if necessary.

First follow-up visit and subsequent course

Frieda stayed home, as instructed, except for her daily visit to Tyrone. She liked Tyrone, but she had a hard time communicating with him in her broken English. He liked her too and offered to bring the medications to her home so that she wouldn't have to come to the hospital every day while she was supposed to be staying off her bad knee.

At Frieda's first follow-up visit with the rheumatologist, the knee was still swollen and a little tender. The doctor, aided by Tyrone, drained the knee again, but the volume of fluid she was able to get from the knee was about half what she had obtained before the onset of treatment. She noted that the sensitivity tests had shown that the germ infecting Frieda's knee was fully sensitive to INH, so she discontinued the EMB, leaving Frieda on INH, RIF, and PZA.

Disease at a Glance: Infectious Arthritis

Who Gets It?

- Anybody

Joint involvement

- Usually a single joint (monoarticular arthritis)
- Usually (not always) very painful, swollen, red, warm

Other Features and Complications

- Fever may or may not be present
- Often rapidly destructive
- Frequently superimposed on another form of arthritis, such as rheumatoid arthritis

Lab Results

- Positive culture of joint fluid
- Blood culture may be positive
- Acute phase reactants (sedimentation rate and C-reactive protein) may be elevated
- Joint fluid often has very high white-cell count

Treatment

- Education
- Joint drainage, usually surgical
- Systemic antibiotics (ATB)
  - Broad-spectrum ATB until organism identified
  - Appropriate specific ATB after organism identified
  - Adequate dose and duration of treatment
- Joint reconstruction surgery (if needed) after the infection is cured

Her knee kept getting better. The swelling had gone down completely by the fifth week of treatment, and the rheumatologist no longer needed to drain fluid from the knee. The X-rays showed only minimal joint damage, and the doctor said that Frieda could return to work on a light schedule.

When she reached the eight-week point, the doctor told her that she was ready to begin the continuation phase. The doctor collected a sputum sample (material coughed up from the respiratory tract) to test for TB germs, reduced the number of drugs to two—INH and a longer-acting form of RIF called rifapentine, or RPT—and reduced the frequency of administration from once daily to once weekly. The sputum sample was negative, and the doctor told Frieda that the continuation phase of treatment would last for 18 weeks, after which she would not need further treatment.

Frieda's Outcome

A few weeks after completing her course of antituberculous therapy, Frieda took stock of her situation with respect to her pending retirement. Because she had lived so frugally, putting away most of her small salary over the years, she was in pretty good shape financially. She would be able to start collecting Social Security in a few more months and would be able to live reasonably comfortably without working regularly. Frieda got rid of her tuberculosis with minimal damage to her knee and never suffered another bout.

Chapter 10

Enteropathic Arthritis, or Inflammatory Bowel Disease

Onset: Rumbling in the Back Passage

Edgar was a fastidious young bachelor. As an accountant, he was the ultimate model of well-organized efficiency. No one in the finance department had a neater desk or a tidier cubicle. Edgar took good care of himself and prided himself that his health was good. His only problems were long-standing constipation and, for the past few months, some aching and stiffness in the wrists and elbows. Sometimes his knees bothered him, but he was able to get reasonable relief by taking two or three ibuprofen capsules a few times daily during such periods.

You can imagine Edgar's embarrassment when, one day, without any warning, he began to have uncontrollable flatulence at irregular but increasingly frequent intervals. These were not just quiet, easily ignored small amounts of rapidly dispersed gas, but great, thunderous, odoriferous expulsions that commanded the attention and overwhelmed the senses of all in the office.

Contrary to the satisfaction that one might reasonably expect from the elimination of large, unwanted volumes of intestinal gas, his bowels were suddenly seized with cramping pains such as he had never experienced. Abandoning dignity, he sprang from his desk chair and, gripping his abdomen, ran for the men's room. It was just down the hall, and he almost made it in time. But just as he was crashing into the lone empty stall, he lost control, and—well, you can imagine the rest.

To Edgar's horror, as if things were not bad enough, he noticed that, mixed in with the unformed bowel movement were large amounts of what appeared to be dark red blood. Now, in addition to the drained sensation that followed his explosive attack of diarrhea, Edgar was frightened. What in the world was going on?

It was not in his nature to procrastinate, and as soon as Edgar was moderately presentable, he asked a coworker to drive him to the local hospital's emergency room. The emergency-room doctor inserted an intravenous line and quickly decided that Edgar needed to be admitted for intravenous fluids and possibly a blood transfusion, as well as evaluation and control of gastrointestinal bleeding.

Edgar's Assessment

Edgar was in the hospital for three days, during which he underwent the most comprehensive set of examinations he had ever experienced. It seemed to Edgar that his every orifice was probed and explored, every blood test was performed, and every X-ray was taken. During a colonoscopy (direct video examination of the colon using a small camera introduced through a flexible tube, called a colonoscope, inserted in the anus), multiple biopsies (tissue specimens) were taken. After all these tests, the doctor, a gastroenterologist, told Edgar that he had Crohn's disease, an inflammatory disease of the intestinal wall, and that he would need to be on medications for it.

The doctor explained to Edgar that his case was somewhat unusual in that Crohn's disease usually starts with abdominal pain, poor appetite, and weight loss rather than bloody diarrhea. Nonetheless, the diagnosis was confirmed by the biopsy. In addition, the doctor thought that the joint pains Edgar had been experiencing might be related to the Crohn's disease. He noted that a form of arthritis, often called enteropathic arthritis or IBD (inflammatory bowel disease) arthritis, is the most common nongastrointestinal complication of Crohn's disease, occurring in about 25 percent of cases. He indicated that it was likely that this arthritis would improve as the inflammatory process in the intestine responded to treatment.

All about Enteropathic Arthritis

Crohn's disease is one of many diseases that can have arthritis as a symptom. Although it is pretty clear in Crohn's disease that the gastrointestinal component is the primary disease, in many other diseases it can be hard to tell whether arthritis or some other feature of the disease is primary. Systemic lupus erythematosus, for example, may start off looking like rheumatoid arthritis or juvenile idiopathic arthritis. Sometimes the primary disease takes awhile to declare itself and leaves doctors scratching their heads until the disease is fully expressed. This can take months in some cases. This rarely happens with Crohn's disease, however.

There are at least two types of enteropathic arthritis. The more common form, which Edgar displayed, affects one or more large joints of the extremities—elbows, wrists, knees, ankles. Less commonly, it can also affect the small joints of the hands, as rheumatoid arthritis does. In some ways, this form of enteropathic arthritis resembles RA, but unlike rheumatoid arthritis, the rheumatoid factor test tends to be negative (see chapter 2). This arthritis features swelling of the affected joint or joints, with stiff-ness, warmth, and tenderness. There is often a tendency for much of the soreness to be around the affected joints, rather than within them, and this is referred to as periarticular inflammation. It usu-ally doesn't cause permanent damage to the joints. Moreover, it tends to be active when the intestinal component of the disease is active and quiet when the intestines are quiet. Good control of the intestinal inflammation of Crohn's disease tends to keep this arthritis in check.

The other type of enteropathic arthritis closely resembles anky-losing spondylitis. It mainly involves the joints of the spine and the sacroiliac joints. In this condition, the inflammatory joint activ-ity does not necessarily parallel that in the intestine. It can cause joint damage similar to that of primary ankylosing spondylitis (as described in chapter 5). People who get this form of enteropathic arthritis often have the HLA-B27 antigen, just as do those who have primary ankylosing spondylitis. This type of arthritis must be treated independently of the intestinal disease, and control of the latter doesn't necessarily help the former, or vice versa.

What is Crohn's disease?

There are basically two types of disease—other than infections—that result from chronic inflammation in the wall of the intes-tines. These are both referred to generically as inflammatory bowel disease, or IBD. Ulcerative colitis, which mainly affects the large intestine, or colon, is one of them, and Crohn's disease, which affects both the small and large intestines, is the other. In Crohn's disease, the inflammation has a particular appearance under the microscope that pathologists call granulomatous inflammation. This type of inflammation, which also occurs in tuberculosis, has more or less round aggregations of cells typically found in chronic inflammation—as distinguished from acute inflammation—and central areas of dead tissue, called central necrosis. Recognizing these granulomatous areas is how pathologists can distinguish

Crohn's disease from ulcerative colitis, which is not characterized by granuloma formation.

Crohn's disease is named after Dr. Burrill B. Crohn, a specialist in gastrointestinal diseases, who described it in 1932 in a paper coauthored with two of his colleagues, Dr. Leon Ginzburg and Dr. Gordon Oppenheimer. All three worked together at Mount Sinai Hospital in New York City. They found and described 14 patients with this form of inflammatory bowel disease. They called it regional ileitis because it most frequently affected the third part of the small intestine, called the ileum. Dr. Crohn initially didn't believe that this disease ever affected the large intestine, but later he became convinced that it could. In fact, it can occur anywhere in the gastrointestinal tract, including the esophagus.

Crohn's disease usually begins in men and women between the ages of 25 and 40. It sometimes even affects children. It is more common in those who live in the Northern Hemisphere, who have relatively higher socioeconomic status, and who smoke. Although Crohn's disease can cause bloody diarrhea, as it did in Edgar's case, it frequently starts with abdominal pain, constipation, and weight loss. Fever is often present. There are some very nasty things that it can do, including the formation of a connection, or fistula, between the lower intestine and the urinary bladder, the vagina, or the skin around the anus, with drainage of bowel contents through this fistulous tract.

What causes Crohn's disease?

Crohn's disease may be associated, at least in some people, with genetically determined immune system abnormalities that allow the intestinal wall to be attacked by bacteria that normally inhabit the intestine. Specifically, in 2001, scientists studying people with Crohn's disease found in the cells of their intestinal wall frequent mutations of the NOD2 gene, one of the genes that controls an early-warning system indicating the presence of bacterial proteins.

This may allow intestinal bacteria, which ordinarily would not be harmful, to attack the intestinal wall and set off the inflammatory mechanisms that cause the disease.

Whether NOD2 mutation is the primary problem or even a significant problem in the mechanism of Crohn's disease is certainly not clear at this time. And it really doesn't directly explain the arthritis, which in Edgar's situation was probably reactive—that is, caused by remote inflammation.

But other causes have been suggested, including viruses—such as the measles virus, for instance—and bacteria not normally found in the intestine. One such bacterium that has come under suspicion is *Mycobacterium paratuberculosis.* Involvement of this type of bacterium, related to the tuberculosis organism, could explain the granulomatous appearance of the intestinal biopsy in Crohn's disease.

The bottom line is that we really don't yet know for sure what causes Crohn's disease, but we strongly suspect that an autoimmune mechanism, possibly such as the one just described, is at the heart of the matter.

What causes enteropathic arthritis?

The non-HLA-B27–related enteropathic arthritis that occurs in Crohn's disease appears to be related to the primary disease (that is, Crohn's) in much the same way that arthritis occurs in systemic lupus erythematosus. It appears to be a part of the disease, in that its activity tends to fluctuate in relation to the activity of the bowel disease. Successful treatment of the bowel disease controls the arthritis as well, just as successful treatment of systemic lupus controls the arthritis of lupus. Its mechanism of disease is unknown.

On the other hand, the HLA-B27-related form of enteropathic arthritis has a more distant relationship with the primary disease. Its activity, as noted previously, fluctuates independently of the bowel disease and may need to be treated as a separate disorder co-occurring with the bowel disease. The mechanism(s) that produce this form of arthritis are unknown as well.

What are the symptoms of enteropathic arthritis?

Since arthritis in these conditions is not generally the primary symptom, you will probably first be diagnosed with one of the two types of enteropathic, or IBD, ailments discussed above (Crohn's disease or ulcerative colitis). If you have been diagnosed with one of these diseases and are also suffering from tender, swollen joints or joint pain, you are likely to have a form of enteropathic arthritis.

Besides arthritis, what are the other complications of Crohn's disease?

Inside the gastrointestinal tract, the two most common complications are intestinal obstruction and fistulous tract formation.

- Intestinal obstruction is an acute emergency requiring hospitalization and often a surgical approach. Symptoms are severe abdominal pain, vomiting, abdominal distension, and no passage of gas via the rectum.

- A fistulous tract is a tunnel that originates in an inflamed portion of the intestine and works its way either to the skin—generally around the anal area—or to the inside of a hollow organ such as the urinary bladder or the vagina. This allows bowel contents to pass through the fistula. If this material gets into the urinary bladder, it is certain to cause an infection in that organ. Such fistulous tracts usually have to be removed surgically.

- Inflammtory bowel disease, allowed to remain active, may lead to intestinal cancer.

Besides arthritis, Crohn's disease may be complicated by skin eruptions, gallstones, liver disease, or eye inflammation. These are not really uncommon, but they are less frequent than enteropathic arthritis. The connection of each of these complications with the underlying gastrointestinal disease remains poorly understood. Genetic factors might play a role, but it is not certain.

Can enteropathic arthritis be prevented?

No preventive measures for Crohn's disease or enteropathic arthritis have been identified, and we do not know of any clear-cut risk factors for this condition. Since so little is understood about the connections between gastrointestinal diseases and their complications, including the link to arthritis, there isn't anything you can do to prevent it. The best approach is to be aware of your body and to visit a physician if you notice anything unusual going on with your digestive system, particularly if it is persistent. And, of course, don't forget to mention any aches or pains you may have noticed over the same period of time.

Can diet help?

One thing that seems certain is that Crohn's disease is not caused by dietary deficiencies or psychological stresses, although the latter may aggravate the disease, as can dietary indiscretions. Thus dietary treatment is not very effective. Still, we generally recommend that people with active inflammatory bowel disease follow a low-residue, low-fiber diet. Details of such a diet are beyond the scope of this book, but the emphasis is on foods that contain little or no insoluble fiber, such as dairy products, clear liquids, pulpless fruit juices and vegetable juices, etc. This may lessen the stress on the intestinal tract by reducing the bulk of material that it has to handle, which may help minimally. More importantly, it is necessary to make sure that the diet is well balanced and has the right mix of vitamins and minerals, and this is especially relevant in the face of significant diarrhea.

Should I exercise if I have enteropathic arthritis?

See chapter 2 for the discussion of exercising with rheumatoid arthritis; the same suggestions apply here.

How common is enteropathic arthritis?

The frequency of enteropathic arthritis associated with Crohn's disease or ulcerative colitis is not well established, but it may occur in approximately 25 percent of the million or so people affected.

Treating Enteropathic Arthritis

Specific treatment of enteropathic arthritis is probably only necessary in those situations where the arthritis is HLA-B27–positive and looks like either reactive arthritis or ankylosing spondylitis (see chapter 5). In the more common form, treatment of the underlying inflammatory bowel disease generally improves the arthritis as well.

Over the years, many medications have been used to treat inflammatory bowel disease, with or without enteropathic arthritis, and several are effective. All of our drug treatments are aimed at reducing the inflammation in the intestinal wall. Some work directly against inflammation by one mechanism or another; others work against presumed causes of inflammation, such as bacterial infection or autoimmunity. The surgeon also has a role in treating some patients.

The current treatment guidelines take into account the location, severity, and level of disease activity as well as the range of complications that are present.

Can Crohn's disease be cured?

Unfortunately, the answer is no. But we can treat it much more successfully now than in the past. We can't cure the arthritis that is often a part of it.

Like many incurable inflammatory diseases, Crohn's disease is usually characterized by periods of activity, called exacerbations or flares, separated by periods of relative quiescence, called remissions.

What factors are considered when choosing a treatment plan?

The treatment plan must address the inflammatory bowel disease as the most important part of the problem, taking into account its severity, activity level, and the complications that are present. If arthritis is present, its type will determine whether this must be treated as a separate problem (the HLA-B27–positive spondyloarthropathy type) or whether treatment of the inflammatory bowel disease is likely to take care of the arthritis as well (the more common, large-joint type that Edgar had).

Edgar's Treatment

Because his disease was very active when he entered the hospital, Edgar was started on the best medication available for quickly reducing inflammation and settling down an acute flare: the corticosteroid prednisone. Edgar immediately began to make great strides, and as his doctor gradually reduced the dose, he began maintenance treatment. Because Edgar didn't have intestinal obstruction or fistulous tracts, the doctor didn't think surgery was necessary at that time. Edgar's joint symptoms responded to the treatment of his Crohn's disease.

Medication

Maintenance drug treatment for Crohn's disease includes the use of an aminosalicylate, and for this, Edgar's doctor prescribed mesalamine. These anti-inflammatory medications can be tolerated for longer periods of time than the corticosteroids. But they are not as strong, and if the disease flares up again as prednisone is discontinued, aminosalicylates might have to be supplemented with other medications, such as the immunosuppressive drugs azathioprine or methotrexate, or the antibiotics metronidazole or ciprofloxacin.

Recently, the very strong anti-inflammatory biologic drug infliximab has been found effective, both in aiding prednisone in the induction of an initial remission and in supplementing the aminosalicylates in maintaining a remission.

What are the side effects of treatment for Crohn's disease with or without arthritis?

All these drugs have multiple side effects that are potentially severe if they aren't discovered early. It's critical that your doctor monitor your treatment closely if you are taking these medications so that any side effects can be detected and steps can be taken to minimize their untoward results.

Prednisone Prednisone probably has a larger variety of potentially serious side effects than any of the other drugs, and that is why we use it sparingly and stop it as soon as we can. It can cause increased susceptibility to infection; weight gain; loss of bone calcium, or osteoporosis; diabetes; high blood pressure; fluid retention; mental and emotional aberrations (running the gamut from simple mood swings through overt psychosis); cataracts; and acne. Generally, however, for short-term use to shut down a flare-up of the disease, most of these would be very unlikely. The big problems with prednisone in Crohn's disease tend to occur if we can't get a person off the drug and onto a reasonable maintenance program.

Mesalamine Mesalamine and other salicylates can cause diarrhea, headache, abdominal pain, flatulence, malaise, fatigue, and nausea. You will probably notice that some of these side effects sound a lot like what Edgar experienced with his initial attack of Crohn's disease. Although none of these is particularly dangerous, any of them could indicate either that the drug is ineffective or that it is causing a side effect. Either way, you would need to stop the drug.

Azathioprine Azathioprine is an immunosuppressive drug that was used extensively in the early days of organ transplantation to prevent immune rejection. We now have much stronger and better—though more toxic—drugs for that purpose, but azathioprine is still used to treat certain autoimmune conditions these days. Its use in Crohn's disease is based on the theory, by no means proven, that autoimmunity plays a role in this condition. Side effects include a low white blood cell count, resulting in reduced resistance to infection; anemia (low red cell count); a low platelet count with increased risk of bleeding; and liver damage.

Azathioprine also has significant drug interactions with allopurinol, a drug used to treat gout; warfarin, an anticoagulant drug used to prevent blood clotting; and blood pressure drugs known as angiotensin-converting enzyme (ACE) inhibitors.

Methotrexate Methotrexate, also used to treat rheumatoid arthritis and certain other rheumatic diseases, can cause anemia, a low white blood cell count with increased susceptibility to infection, low platelet count with increased risk of bleeding, liver damage, pneumonia, nausea, and drowsiness (see chapter 2 for more information about methotrexate).

Antibiotics Metronidazole can cause neurological symptoms, including tingling and burning sensations in the extremities (peripheral neuropathy) and seizures. It also can interact adversely with warfarin, the sedative phenobarbital, and phenytoin, an antiseizure medication.

Ciprofloxacin can cause seizures, bloody diarrhea, tendon ruptures, and allergic rashes. It can interact adversely with warfarin and certain other drugs.

TNF-Alpha Inhibitors Infliximab is a new biological drug that suppresses inflammation by inhibiting the important mediator tumor necrosis factor-alpha, or TNF-alpha (see chapter 2). It is generally given intravenously, but there is interest in its effects on Crohn's disease when administered by mouth. Infliximab can reduce resistance to infection and even lower the white blood cell count. There is also some evidence that infliximab can increase the likelihood of developing lymphoma, a type of malignancy affecting the lymph nodes. Some people have allergic reactions to infliximab, and occasionally people have had lupuslike reactions, with rash, arthritis, and positive tests for antinuclear antibodies. People with demyelinating diseases—which attack the myelin coating that insulates and protects nerve fibers—of the central nervous system, such as multiple sclerosis, can be made worse by infliximab, and the drug should be avoided or used with great caution in this setting.

What is the role of surgery?

There are some situations where surgery is necessary on an emergency basis. If the intestine perforates, releasing intestinal contents into the abdominal cavity, that is a disaster that quickly leads to peritonitis, sepsis, and death unless emergency surgery is performed. Intestinal obstruction that does not resolve with the placement of a tube into the intestine may also require surgery. Finally, persistent activity of the disease in spite of drug treatment may require a surgical approach.

If an operation is necessary, the surgeon generally removes the inflamed section of the intestine. Depending on how much intestine has to be removed, this can have long-term consequences for nutrition. The small intestine is normally 12 to 20 feet in length. If a large portion has to be removed (leaving less than 5 feet of small intestine if the colon has to be removed or less than 2 feet of small intestine if the colon is preserved), this is called short bowel syndrome, and the patient may need total parenteral nutrition— that is, all nutrition given intravenously. Sometimes the surgical procedure requires the temporary or permanent rerouting of the end of the intestine to the surface of the abdomen—colostomy or ileostomy, depending on the part of the intestine at the orifice—and the use of a bag to collect the fecal material.

What is the status of Crohn's disease research?

A great deal of research is under way, both as to the basic mechanisms of Crohn's disease as well as the effectiveness of treatment. Since the disease was recognized just over 75 years ago, it is a relative baby among diseases. There is still plenty we don't know about it, including how the arthritis is produced. Controversy exists about some aspects of it as well.

Dr. William Sandborn, an expert in the study of inflammatory bowel disease, has pointed out that Dr. Richard Farmer proposed the first classification of Crohn's disease from his study of 615 patients at the Cleveland Clinic in the mid-1970s. This classification was based mainly on the anatomic location of bowel inflammation: small intestine, 29 percent; large intestine, 27 percent; or both, 41 percent—with the last group having the most complications.

Another classification, proposed by Dr. David Sachar at Mount Sinai Hospital in New York about a decade later, further subdivided 770 surgical patients with Crohn's disease into those with perforating disease (20 percent) and nonperforating disease (80 percent). But by the time you follow the patients for ten years, the 80 percent with no complications is down to about 20 percent.

What does all this mean? Over time, increasing numbers of patients get complications, many of which require surgery. About 40 percent of the patients come to surgery within two years after diagnosis, and this is about half of the patients who ever undergo surgery.

When Edgar's doctor explained this to him, he observed, "That sounds like there is probably an operation in my future."

"Given today's technology, that's probably true," agreed his doctor. "But new medical treatments are being developed all the time, and there is great hope that the present discouraging results can be improved upon."

Edgar's Response to Treatment

Edgar did quite well over the next few months. He tolerated the prednisone well and eventually was able to get off of it completely. His arthritis resolved as he got his Crohn's disease under control. He continued to take mesalamine and tolerated it well. He had occasional gastrointestinal symptoms—just enough not to forget that he had Crohn's disease—but in reality, it was not entirely clear whether the gas he continued to have from time to time originated from the disease or the treatment.

What happens if treatment stops working?

The approach described above is the currently accepted protocol for treatment of this condition. Surgical removal of portions of the intestine resistant to medical treatment is the ultimate treatment available at this time.

What to Expect

For the acute episode, drugs—especially prednisone—generally work pretty well. Most people get a favorable response initially. But Crohn's disease is a chronic condition, and it tends to relapse after periods of remission, even in the face of fairly aggressive treatment. Unfortunately, none of the drugs we have now can keep the disease in remission permanently, and we usually need to go back to prednisone, either alone or in combination with one or more other drugs, from time to time to restore order. If the disease becomes intractable and doesn't respond to drug therapy, then we need to call the surgeon.

With respect to enteropathic arthritis, generally no specific antiarthritic treatment is necessary, because the arthritis usually responds to successful treatment for active bowel disease. A flare-up of arthritis might actually be a pretty good indicator that the bowel disease is beginning to reactivate, even though recognizable bowel symptoms may not have appeared. On the other hand, if you have

Disease at a Glance: Enteropathic Arthritis

Who Gets It?

- More common in women than men
- More common in Caucasians than in African-Americans
- Family history often positive
- About 250,000 Americans affected (25 percent of those with Crohn's disease, of which arthritis is the most common complication)

Joint Involvement

- Enteropathic arthritis tends to affect a few joints on the same side of the body
- Inflammation may develop more around the joints than within them, but it can be destructive
- Ankylosing spondylitis occurs in some patients

Other Features and Complications

- Fistula formation
- Intestinal obstruction
- Intestinal perforation

Lab Results

- Acute-phase reactants (sedimentation rate and C-reactive protein) elevated
- HLA-B27 positive in patients with spondylitis
- Negative blood test for rheumatoid factor

Treatment

- General
  - Adequate rest
  - Appropriate exercise
  - Low-residue, low-fiber diet
  - Education

(continued)

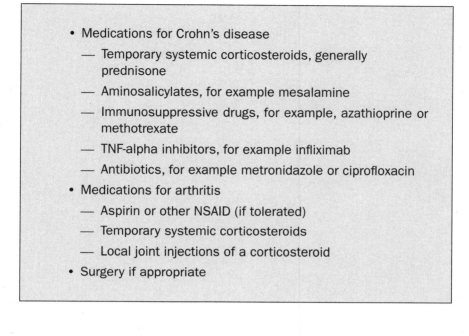

- Medications for Crohn's disease
  — Temporary systemic corticosteroids, generally prednisone
  — Aminosalicylates, for example mesalamine
  — Immunosuppressive drugs, for example, azathioprine or methotrexate
  — TNF-alpha inhibitors, for example infliximab
  — Antibiotics, for example metronidazole or ciprofloxacin
- Medications for arthritis
  — Aspirin or other NSAID (if tolerated)
  — Temporary systemic corticosteroids
  — Local joint injections of a corticosteroid
- Surgery if appropriate

the ankylosing spondylitis–like arthritis with your Crohn's disease, the activity of the arthritis will not necessarily parallel that of the bowel disease and the arthritis will need to be treated as a separate condition.

Edgar's Outcome

Edgar's ultimate outcome is not yet known. His Crohn's disease is not cured, and he continues to have minor flare-ups requiring periodic adjustment of his treatment. It is probable that sometime in the next few years, he will require surgery unless new approaches to this disease are developed.

Considering all that had happened, Edgar found it difficult to maintain his former level of formality and aloofness at work. This was a big step for him. His coworker Miss Perkins—Twyla—began to accompany him on his regular follow-up visits to the doctor, and on one such occasion, about a year after the dramatic onset of Edgar's symptoms, the doctor noticed that she was sporting a spectacular diamond ring on her left fourth finger.

Chapter 11

Polymyalgia Rheumatica

Onset: A Bolt from the Blue

Jed was lying in bed on a wintry morning, enjoying the warmth and musing over a conversation that he'd overheard the day before at the senior center where he volunteered to help other retired older folks with their taxes each year. His wife, Elsie, was still sleeping next to him, but he decided that it was time to get up and get ready for his day at the senior center. He rolled over, but when he sat on the edge of the bed, he knew he was in trouble. Every muscle in his body was sore, and he was stiff as a board. As Jed stood up, his whole pelvis felt as if it were on fire. His hips didn't want to move, and his thighs felt unbearably heavy.

He finally managed to get to the bathroom. Raising his arms to take off his pajama top took tremendous effort and provoked pain throughout the shoulder regions. Jed slipped on his glasses and looked himself over in the mirror. Nothing appeared to be amiss; there was no swelling in the shoulders or the knees. But what in the world was going on?

Jed decided to take a shower to see if that would help. He turned on the water as hot as he could stand it. He noticed that his hands were not stiff or sore, and he had no difficulty turning on the faucets.

He stood under the steaming water and slowly began to loosen up a little. The heat felt good, and some of the soreness seemed to get a little better. But as soon as Jed stepped out of the shower, the soreness and stiffness returned with a vengeance. It was even hard to shave because his shoulders were so sore. He took three aspirin.

Jed sat at the breakfast table, but he really didn't feel like making the effort to brew coffee, unload the dishwasher (one of his morning tasks), go out and get the paper, or pour his cereal. About a half hour had gone by since he'd taken the aspirin, but he felt no better. When Elsie joined him and saw that he was suffering, she called the doctor's office. Jed limped to the car. He felt exhausted by the time they got to the doctor's office, and the soreness was even worse.

Jed's Assessment

The doctor questioned Jed about his symptoms. Then he asked whether Jed had experienced any headache or visual symptoms. He examined Jed thoroughly, paying particular attention to his temples. Jed had no soreness in those areas, one of the few parts of his body that didn't hurt.

When the doctor had finished the exam, he sat with Jed and Elsie and said, "Jed, I think you have a relatively common rheumatic condition called polymyalgia rheumatica; we call it PMR for short."

The doctor felt comfortable treating patients with this disease because, even though he was not a rheumatologist, he knew how to treat it, and he knew that Jed's response to treatment would likely be considered miraculous by the elderly couple.

He wanted to confirm the diagnosis with some laboratory tests. In the meantime, he told Jed that he wanted to start him on low-dose prednisone. He explained that Jed's response to this corticosteroid drug would also help confirm the diagnosis.

All about Polymyalgia Rheumatica

Polymyalgia rheumatica is a condition that causes pain and stiffness in the muscles, particularly around the shoulders and hips. It typically begins suddenly, and it mainly affects people past the age of 50. PMR generally doesn't affect the joints; therefore it is really not a form of arthritis in most people, although some folks get knee swelling with it. Also, it generally doesn't cause pain around the hands, wrists, feet, or ankles.

PMR was considered a disease in England before it was recognized here in the United States, and as diseases go, it was described rather recently. Dr. William Bruce first called it senile rheumatic gout in 1888, but it is obviously not gout. Other names for the condition included rhizomelic pseudoarthrosis, humeroscapular periarthrosis, and anarthritic rheumatoid syndrome. It was not until 1957 that the name polymyalgia rheumatica was given to it by Dr. H. Stuart Barber.

What causes PMR?

Like many of the rheumatic diseases, the cause of polymyalgia rheumatica is unknown. The leading candidates for causation are infection or autoimmunity, but there is not really much evidence for either one. Some years ago, there was interest in the theory that an infectious agent carried by birds might be the cause, because many people who got PMR had pet birds in their houses. Although this was never disproved, it wasn't proven either, and the idea, though interesting, is not accepted by most authorities. Recent wisdom is that the pain of PMR is caused by synovitis, which is inflammation of joint membranes; or by bursitis, which is inflammation of the fluid sacs, or bursas, that cushion and protect muscles from rubbing underlying tissues or bones.

What are the symptoms of PMR?

The typical features of PMR are pain and stiffness in the muscles of the shoulders and pelvic region. It often, but not always, starts suddenly, just as it did in Jed's case.

Is PMR genetic?

There does seem to be a genetic component to PMR. It is associated with one of the genetically determined white-cell antigens, called HLA-DR4. The gene for this antigen is also found in many patients with rheumatoid factor–positive rheumatoid arthritis. The HLA-DR4 gene seems to be one of the determinants of autoimmunity.

Does PMR predispose me to other diseases?

PMR has an association with a much more serious condition called giant cell arteritis, or GCA, an inflammation of arteries' inner walls. It primarily affects arteries in the head, including the temporal arteries, which are located just under the skin in front of the upper part of the ears. If you put your finger there lightly, you can feel your temporal artery pulse.

GCA occurs in a small percentage of people with PMR. It is painful and causes headache and tenderness in the temporal regions. But the greatest significance of GCA is that it can cause sudden and irreversible vision loss. That's why the doctor asked Jed about headache and visual disturbances and felt his temporal arteries.

If you display any signs of GCA, your doctor will likely start you immediately on a larger dose of prednisone. He might also order a temporal artery biopsy to confirm the diagnosis. The arterial walls of people with GCA have a unique appearance under the microscope, the most characteristic feature of which is the presence of large cells with multiple nuclei, called giant cells. High-dose prednisone, started early enough and continued for about six weeks, usually is adequate to prevent blindness.

GCA can also cause some other nasty complications, such as gangrene (tissue death due to impaired blood supply) of a portion of the scalp or tongue, a strokelike condition, and other symptoms resulting from a lack of blood flow to organs or tissues served by the affected arteries.

Occasionally GCA appears late in someone being treated for PMR, usually if the prednisone has been reduced or discontinued prematurely. But with careful monitoring, the onset of GCA late in the treatment for PMR is unlikely.

Can PMR be prevented?

There is no known method for preventing PMR.

Can diet help?

Diet provides no known benefit in PMR.

Should I exercise if I have PMR?

A good exercise program for cardiovascular fitness and muscle stretching and strengthening is beneficial in PMR. The level of exercise should be age-appropriate and take into account any known heart or neurological disease. A rule of thumb for determining maximal exercise capacity is that level of exercise that produces a heart rate of 220/minute minus age in years. You should not exceed about 75 percent of the maximal calculated rate. For example, if you are 65 years old, your level of exercise should not exceed that which produces a heart rate of 75 percent of 220 minus 65, which is 116 per minute. Check with your doctor to see if there are any reasons you should not do this.

How common is PMR?

In the United States, the frequency has been reported to be 52.5 cases per 100,000 persons aged 50 years and older.

Treating Polymyalgia Rheumatica

Polymyalgia rheumatica is nearly always satisfactorily treated with prednisone, and no other treatment appears to work as well. The dose depends on whether the patient has any signs of temporal arteritis. Generally, if no signs are present, the starting dose can be 15 to 20 milligrams of prednisone daily. Once the symptoms have been controlled, the dose can be lowered gradually to 5 to 7.5 milligrams daily. Doctors aren't in complete agreement on how high the dose should be if there are signs of temporal arteritis, but 40 to 60 milligrams daily for six weeks is probably the right range, followed by gradual reduction to a daily range of 5 to 10 milligrams.

Can PMR be cured?

This is one of the few rheumatic diseases that adequate treatment can regularly put in complete remission. It may take five to ten years, but once it occurs, prednisone can be tapered and discontinued.

What factors are considered when choosing a treatment plan?

The major considerations are preexisting conditions that may be exacerbated by prednisone, such as diabetes, hypertension, osteoporosis, cataracts, and infection. Prednisone can still be used, but with caution and close observation.

Jed's Treatment

Jed's doctor prescribed him a low dosage of prednisone: 15 milligrams daily. He asked Jed to return in a week. But Jed didn't listen. He waited a day before starting the prednisone, thinking that a good night's rest might just clear up the whole thing. But he was wrong. If anything, he felt worse the next morning, and as soon as he got up, he took the prednisone. By noon, he felt somewhat better, and by the next morning, he felt completely normal. He kept taking the prednisone daily, and by the time he returned to the doctor's office a week later, he felt as though he'd never been sick a day in his life.

The doctor told Jed that the tests for rheumatoid arthritis, lupus, and other conditions had all been negative, but the red-cell sedimentation rate was markedly elevated to 120 millimeters per hour. In PMR and most other inflammatory conditions, there are elevated levels of proteins in the blood called acute-phase reactants. These affect the rate at which red cells settle from blood on standing. This rate, measured in a special tube, is called the sedimentation rate, and it is normally expressed in millimeters per hour. This is characteristic of PMR, and the rapid, complete response to low-dose prednisone is also very typical.

Jed's Response to Treatment

Jed did very well on the prednisone, but the doctor had mentioned that he might have side effects if he took it for too long. Prednisone controlled his symptoms, and side effects were minimal, including some thinning of the skin and easy bruising.

How long do I have to take prednisone?

Experience has shown that PMR patients like Jed probably need to take prednisone for at least two years, and perhaps for as long as ten.

Although it is likely that you can reduce the dose almost immediately to between 5 and 7.5 milligrams daily, going below that in the first two years almost invariably causes a relapse. After that, your doctor may try reducing the dose every six months, as long as no symptoms recur. Eventually you should be able to stop the prednisone altogether, although there are some people who need to take it indefinitely.

What are the side effects of prednisone?

Prednisone side effects tend to be related to dose and duration. That means that the higher the dose or the longer you take it, the more likely you are to experience side effects. In PMR cases, you tend to see the effects of prolonged treatment, but not those produced by high doses. Over time you will see some thinning of the skin and some superficial bruising, and you may have a tendency to gain weight and to lose calcium from the bones, which is called osteoporosis. Some people on long-term prednisone develop cataracts even when the dose is low.

Other side effects include hypertension, "moon face," abnormal redistribution of body fat to the trunk and away from the extremities, purple stretch marks on the abdomen, susceptibility to infection, and diabetes. These are more common in people on higher doses of prednisone, but they are not unknown even at low doses taken for a long time. Some people even have psychiatric disturbances induced by prednisone, generally restricted to mood swings but sometimes more severe, and overt psychoses brought on by prednisone are not unknown.

Fortunately, most of these conditions are rare and they are also mostly reversible upon discontinuing the drug. They don't necessarily reverse rapidly, however.

Are there alternatives to prednisone in treating PMR?

There were high hopes a number of years ago, particularly in England, that the nonsteroidal anti-inflammatory drugs, or NSAIDs, might prove effective against PMR, but they didn't. Furthermore, they provided no protection against GCA. There has been experimentation with drugs such as methotrexate that might allow the prescribing physician to minimize the dose of prednisone, but results have been disappointing.

Disease at a Glance: Polymyalgia Rheumatica

Who Gets It?
- Onset generally after age 50
- Women affected more commonly than men
- Sudden onset typical

Joint involvement
- Predominantly affects muscle (typically the muscles of the shoulders and hips)
- Synovitis in knees sometimes occurs

Other Features and Complications
- Giant cell (temporal) arteritis may be associated with PMR

Lab Results
- Very high sedimentation rate
- Negative blood test for rheumatoid factor

Treatment
- General
  — Education
- Medications
  — Prednisone

What to Expect

If you have PMR, you can expect that after a period of treatment with prednisone (the exact length of which can't be accurately predicted), you will be able to get off treatment.

Will I be disabled?

PMR does not cause permanent disability.

Jed's Outcome

Jed continued his prednisone, and within a month he was able to get the dose down to 5 milligrams per day. He continued to feel well. His doctor put him on supplemental calcium and vitamin D to ward off osteoporosis and checked him frequently for diabetes and hypertension. It took several tries over the next five years, but Jed was finally able to get himself totally off prednisone without relapsing. His vision remained intact, and he and Elsie enjoyed their retirement.

Chapter 12

Fibromyalgia

Onset: A Pain in the Neck

Mabel was seated—it felt more like rooted—in her accustomed position in front of her office computer, scrolling through spreadsheet after spreadsheet of numbers in small print. It was already eight-thirty at night, and Mabel was getting bleary-eyed after 12 solid hours of work. It didn't help that she had broken her computer glasses and was working with her bifocals on. This made it necessary for her to tilt her head back to see the screen clearly. Her neck was sore, and when she stretched, she noticed that her shoulders were sore as well. Her upper back was burning with pain, especially around the shoulder blades. Her head ached. She felt miserable, not unlike the way she had felt the last couple of weeks at the end of each day. She looked forward to getting home, sipping a glass of wine, luxuriating in a warm bath, and hitting the sack early. She would feel better tomorrow.

When Mabel got home, the wine hit the spot and the bath was soothing. During the night, however, she was unable to find a comfortable position in bed. She tossed and turned. She tried lying on one side, then the other, with and without a pillow. She took three aspirins. She tried rubbing her neck. She put a heating pad she had inherited from her mother on her neck, and then a plastic bag full of ice cubes, both to no avail. Finally, around three in the morning, she got up and turned on the TV, figuring that pure boredom would put her to sleep. But she continued to hurt.

Despite her discomfort, she did manage to doze off a few times, and, as it happened, she was snoozing on the sofa in front of the TV when her alarm began beeping at six o'clock. As Mabel struggled to regain consciousness, her pain felt much worse than the night before. This had never happened to her. Normally, a night of rest would ease the pain. Then she recalled that she had not gotten much rest that night. No wonder she felt so bad. She decided to stay home from work that day to see whether she would improve with rest.

That night Mabel felt even worse. She really didn't sleep at all. The next day, she had pain in all the previous locations, but in addition, her knees ached, and she was sore around the brim of the pelvis. She was 34 years old but she felt as if she were 94, and she didn't like it. She swallowed a few more aspirins and called her internist.

Mabel's Assessment

After Mabel recounted the story of the last few days, the doctor asked her many questions about her joints and muscles. Were the joints swollen? Were they stiff? Could she move them through the full range of motion? Were the muscles weak? Did they look swollen or shrunken? Were they tender to the touch? Had any of these symptoms ever occurred before? Was she taking any new medications? Mabel had to admit that similar symptoms had occurred before, but they had never lasted this long or been this severe. The doctor asked about her sleep habits and about her exercise activities. Mabel acknowledged that she sometimes had trouble getting to sleep, especially the last few nights, and that she lived a fairly sedentary lifestyle. She was always tired, and she had become somewhat stout.

The doctor then performed a physical examination, placing his hands on Mabel's shoulders from behind and probing along the top of the shoulders with one finger, looking for tender spots. He soon found one, and Mabel exclaimed, "Yikes! Do you have to do that?" She was about to complain some more, when he found another spot along the inner margin of the left shoulder blade, producing a bolt of pain that rendered her temporarily speechless, but she soon regained her composure and continued rattling off a fusillade of complaints.

By the time the doctor finished examining her, he had found another dozen or so tender points. His conclusion: fibromyalgia.

Mabel was unconvinced. How could he be so sure without doing any tests?

The doctor explained that he did plan to perform some tests, but they would be mainly to rule out some low-probability conditions that mimic fibromyalgia.

All about Fibromyalgia

Fibromyalgia is a painful condition that affects muscles rather than joints. So technically it's not a form of arthritis. It's a clinical diagnosis based on the history and physical findings, which researchers have grouped into a set of diagnostic criteria. Blood tests are all normal in fibromyalgia, and X-rays show very little as well.

What causes fibromyalgia?

Strictly speaking, we don't know. The most popular theory is that muscle tightness causes fibromyalgia. Certainly that seems reasonable, since muscle tightness is clearly a part of the syndrome. If, for whatever reason—for example, sitting for hours in front of a computer—a person's muscles tighten up and remain that way for any length of time, the muscles eventually become fatigued and start to ache. The natural reaction to this is to hold the painful area immobile to reduce the pain. Doing so requires contracting the muscles in the area, but this leads to further local muscle fatigue and pain. It's a vicious cycle. The expenditure of energy results in more generalized fatigue, one of the most common features of fibromyalgia.

As far as we have been able to determine, however, there is no underlying physical muscle abnormality in fibromyalgia, even though that's the source of the pain. There have been many studies of muscle biopsies, using the regular microscope, the electron microscope, and nuclear magnetic resonance (technology similar to that used in MRI, which measures some electrophysiological characteristics of muscle), without any consistent demonstration of abnormalities. Muscle metabolism appears to be normal, and there is no damage to muscle cells, as there is in polymyositis, an inflammatory condition of muscle in which muscle cells are destroyed.

There was a famous study conducted with medical students a couple of decades ago. Two groups of students—the experimental group and the control group—spent several nights in a sleep lab. Those in the experimental group were automatically awakened every time they reached a certain level of sleep called REM (short for rapid eye movement) sleep, which correlates with dreaming. Those in the control group were not awakened from REM sleep. The first group of students developed symptoms of fibromyalgia, while those in the second group did not. This led to the concept that sleep disturbance may play a role in causing fibromyalgia.

Are there other causes of fibromyalgia-like symptoms?

Other conditions sometimes present with symptoms similar to fibromyalgia:

- Hypothyroidism (low thyroid function) has a typical symptom profile, including fatigue, weight gain, a sensation of coldness, hoarseness, dry skin, thinning hair, and muscle pain. The hormonal condition can be diagnosed by way of a simple blood test.

- Polymyalgia rheumatica (see chapter 11) is also characterized by muscle pain. In addition, it includes stiffness and abnormal blood tests, and mainly occurs in people above the age of 50.

- Sometimes fibromyalgialike symptoms occur as a side effect of the so-called statin drugs used to treat high cholesterol. This seemed unlikely in Mabel's case, since she wasn't taking any of these drugs.

What are the symptoms of fibromyalgia?

One of the main characteristics of fibromyalgia is the presence of tender points at some or all of the following 18 specific locations:

- Back of the neck (two points)
- Sides of the neck (two points)
- Tops of the shoulders (two points)
- Front of the shoulders (two points)
- Inner borders of the shoulder blades (two points)
- Outer sides of the elbows (two points)
- Brim of the pelvis (two points)
- Sides of the hips (two points)
- Inner margins of the knees (two points)

Tenderness in at least 11 points, together with a history of widespread pain, fulfills the criteria for the diagnosis of fibromyalgia. In Mabel's case, all 18 points were tender. Other suggestive symptoms are sleep disturbance, fatigue, anxiety, and headache, all of which Mabel claimed to have.

How do you know there is no arthritis in fibromyalgia?

There are no consistent joint abnormalities in fibromyalgia, and such abnormalities are required for the diagnosis of arthritis. The joints do not swell, and they are not inflamed. There is no joint damage, even in people who have symptoms of fibromyalgia for many years.

The neck is commonly involved in fibromyalgia. X-rays often show straightening of the normal curvature of the cervical spine, but this appears to be due to excessive tightness of the neck muscles. The intervertebral joints and disks tend to have a normal appearance.

People with true arthritis sometimes have fibromyalgia as well, but the fibromyalgic symptoms and the arthritic symptoms are easily distinguished from each other. This is true even when both conditions are actively painful at the same time.

What is the relationship between fibromyalgia and chronic fatigue syndrome?

There's no easy answer to this question. Fibromyalgia and chronic fatigue syndrome are both clinical conditions of unknown cause, and although there is some overlap of symptoms between the two—for example, both have prominent fatigue—they are not exactly the same. Chronic fatigue syndrome, sometimes abbreviated as CFS, was originally believed to be caused by chronic infection with Epstein-Barr virus, the bug that causes mononucleosis. This relationship, however, did not pan out consistently, and some experts have postulated that CFS is a form of fibromyalgia in which the fatigue is more prominent than the pain. Some physicians don't believe that either condition exists as a specific disease entity and prefer to consider both as merely being out of sorts. Severely out of sorts, you might say.

Is fibromyalgia genetic?

There is no evidence for a genetic component in fibromyalgia.

Does fibromyalgia predispose me to other diseases?

People with fibromyalgia sometimes have symptoms of depression. It is not clear whether the depression causes the fibromyalgia or vice versa.

Can fibromyalgia be prevented?

The best preventive measures for fibromyalgia are to get adequate rest and exercise regularly. Swimming is a very good general exercise for people who tend toward fibromyalgia.

Can diet help?

There is no credible evidence that fibromyalgia responds positively to dietary measures.

Should I exercise if I have fibromyalgia?

It's very important to stretch your muscles if you have fibromyalgia. As noted above, swimming is a very good general exercise. You should swim two to three times weekly in a heated pool for at least a half hour per session. You have to stay with it, though, and it may take 6 to 12 weeks to get the full benefit. If you don't have access to a place to swim, such as the local Y, or if you try it and don't get any benefit, ask your doctor about a more formal physical therapy program including stretching and strengthening exercises focused on the most painful areas.

How common is fibromyalgia?

I don't know of any good statistics, but it is very common. If we define it strictly, according to the criteria mentioned previously, it is less common but still relatively frequent. And doctors recognize that many of their patients don't quite meet the formal criteria but have basically the same process going on. In fact, there seems to be a continuum of severity of fibromyalgia that has no exact cut-off point at 11 tender points. Some people with essentially the same condition may have only 10 tender points. If they don't have fibromyalgia, then what do they have? In my opinion, I would contend that they have fibromyalgia, because in all other ways they appear to have it.

Treating Fibromyalgia

Because we really don't know the cause of fibromyalgia and have only some unproven theories about the mechanisms involved, treatment is pretty empirical, based on common sense and trial and error rather than science. In my experience, the most beneficial treatment is a combination of adequate rest and active exercise—both stretching and strengthening of the muscle groups involved. Talk to your doctor about appropriate activities. The key is to choose a regimen and stick with it, as results generally take six to eight weeks to reach their peak.

Can fibromyalgia be cured?

There's no cure for fibromyalgia, but patients generally respond well to treatment. If you have fibromyalgia, it is important to keep yourself in good condition with regular physical activity, such as swimming. If you do, the symptoms will be less likely to come back. You can probably stop using a sleep aid after a few weeks, but you may need it periodically to help you get a good night's rest.

Fibromyalgia symptoms may recur at times of stress, either emotional or physical. If you continue your regular exercise program, the symptoms shouldn't be as bad. In such circumstances, your doctor may resume sleep-aid use (if you were taking it before) and perhaps prescribe the muscle relaxant cyclobenzaprine along with it. But overall, the most important things you can do are to keep in good physical condition with your exercise program, maintain your weight in a healthy range, and get adequate rest.

That's not bad advice for anyone, whether they have fibromyalgia or not.

What factors are considered when choosing a treatment plan?

It is important for your doctor to consider the location of fibromyalgic pain, because the exercise program must address the part of the body that hurts. It is also important that you work with him or her to recognize activities that aggravate the problem and attempt to modify them. The treatment must address any sleep problems that can be identified.

Mabel's Treatment

Mabel liked and respected her doctor, and she resolved to do what he recommended. She immediately had her prescription for the sleep aid temazepam (see below) filled, and she signed up for swimming lessons at the local YMCA.

Medication

If you are not sleeping well, your doctor can give you something to help you sleep. Temazepam is a relatively effective medication for this and usually doesn't leave a person groggy the next morning. In the best of all worlds, you shouldn't need sleep assistance once your exercise regimen really becomes effective.

Muscle-relaxing medications may also be useful in fibromyalgia, and we have a number of them to select from. My favorite is cyclobenzaprine. It can give fairly rapid relief, but it tends to make some people drowsy, to the point where it can become unsafe to drive while taking this medication.

Another drug often used for fibromyalgia is doxepin, an antidepressant that may also help with sleep. Many physicians believe that depression plays a role in the genesis of fibromyalgia, and certainly people who have the condition for any length of time are prone to become depressed, perhaps another vicious cycle.

A lot of other remedies for fibromyalgia have been tried, and that's what often happens in conditions where recommended treatments don't always work. It is probably better to stick to mainline therapies initially and give them a chance before branching out into the Never-Never Land of unproven treatments.

Other treatments

If you go to the Web and search for fibromyalgia or the old term for it, fibrositis, you will find all sorts of things, some based on bizarre reasoning, others based on no reasoning at all. An example is guaifenesin, an over-the-counter medicine normally used as an expectorant cough medicine. In the case of guaifenesin, the rationale, as I understand it, is that since the drug reduces the viscosity of upper respiratory secretions, this anti-viscous effect may apply to muscle as well and get things flowing better. There is no evidence that this occurs. Most such remedies are harmless, but there is no data to support their use other than anecdotal testimonials, which have not been rigorously tested.

Mabel's Response to Treatment

To Mabel's surprise, she actually enjoyed her sessions at the Y and began to look forward to them. She got a new prescription for computer glasses from her optometrist and no longer had to cock her neck into an uncomfortable position in order to see her computer screen at work. And she found that the quality of her sleep was greatly improved by taking temazepam at bedtime.

Remarkably, there was also a gradual improvement in her pain. It was so slow that she almost didn't notice it. But by the time of her next appointment, two months later, she was feeling much better, had lost ten pounds, and no longer felt so fatigued. She recounted all this to the doctor. He was glad to hear it and was impressed, among other things, with her leaner appearance.

What happens if the treatment stops working?

If the treatment worked at first and no longer does, look for changes in your activities or stress level. Usually it's not hard to find what changed. If the treatment never worked, it's back to the drawing board. Never forget, however, that even though fibromyalgia is painful, it doesn't cause permanent damage anywhere in the body.

What to Expect

Usually, once a patient diligently follows a beneficial exercise program and modifies her other activities, any relapses prove to be related to some failure to continue the program. Restoring the appropriate activities tends to take care of it. Occasional flare-ups are the norm, but these usually can be handled without great difficulty.

Is fibromyalgia disabling?

Fibromyalgia may be painful, but it does not damage the painful areas. Think of it like a headache. Headaches are very painful, but in most cases, when they subside, there is no residual damage from them. Many painful conditions can be permanently harmful to the body—rheumatoid arthritis, for example. Fibromyalgia is not one of them.

Mabel's Outcome

Mabel continued her exercise program. Her computer glasses took the stress off her neck while she was working and greatly increased her level of comfort. She also found a pillow made of memory foam and designed to relieve neck pain. This helped her to sleep better, and she continues to do well.

Disease at a Glance: Fibromyalgia

Who Gets It?
- Women affected more often than men
- Very common condition
- Worse with stress

Joint Involvement
- Painful muscles, generally in the upper back and the posterior neck
- Tender (trigger) points in typical locations
- Joints not involved

Other Features and Complications
- Frequent headaches
- Sleep disturbances
- Irritable bowel not uncommon
- Straightening of normal curvature in the neck's cervical spine

Lab Results
- No consistent lab abnormalities

Treatment
- General
  — Adequate rest
  — Appropriate exercise (active rather than passive)
  — Education
- Medications
  — Aspirin or other NSAID
  — Muscle-relaxing medications, such as cyclobenzaprine
  — On rare occasions, local tender point injections of corticosteroid or lidocaine

Conclusion

So there you have it—a distillation of what I have learned over the years about arthritis and similar conditions. During my years in practice, many things have changed in rheumatology: the recognition of a whole category of arthritis that had not previously been differentiated from rheumatoid arthritis—the spondyloarthropathies; recognition that methotrexate could be used safely to treat a variety of rheumatic diseases; the development of a whole new class of very effective biologic drugs, TNF-alpha inhibitors, developed from recombinant DNA technology and directed rationally at molecular targets identified by painstaking research; and drugs that essentially take gout off the table as a major arthritic problem.

One of the most amazing things has been the development and refinement of joint replacement surgery. Gone are the days when we used to say, "If you want to keep a secret from an orthopedic surgeon, publish it!" Many of the best and brightest medical school graduates now train in orthopedics. That specialty has come of age, and it's wonderful to see what they can do for our patients by replacing a bad hip, knee, or shoulder.

I believe that we are poised to begin to see the fruits of the unraveling of the human genome, and that we are about to see a revolution in diagnosis and treatment. A new understanding of how diseases evolve and how diseases should be better classified will unfold. Many surgical procedures and potentially dangerous medical treatments may eventually become obsolete.

It would be nice if all this could be done within the context of a great cost reduction in health care, better preventive care, and universal access to the best care. That may be a little too much to hope for in the near future, but it's coming some day!

Appendix 1

Participation in Clinical Trials

Should I Participate in a Clinical Trial Testing an Experimental Therapy?

It is very important for the advancement of science and patient care that many fully informed people are willing to volunteer for clinical trials. Everyone owes these participants gratitude for their sacrifice. But no one can be forced to take part, and it is unethical and morally indefensible for anyone to be experimented on without his or her knowledge or consent.

Volunteering for a clinical trial is highly worthwhile if the trial is well designed and is examining an important issue. Such trials are necessary to bring new treatments into general use. Your rheumatologist can help you technically evaluate a particular trial that might interest you. You need to realize, however, that the essence of research is finding an answer where none exists, so there is always an element of risk in such trials that goes beyond the risk that exists in everyday medicine. Only you can decide to take that risk, and you can't make a good decision unless you know what risks are thought to exist. Not only is there the risk that the new treatment might not work, but also that it might actually be dangerous in previously unsuspected ways. There are several protections built into well-designed studies that reduce the likelihood of injury to study participants, but injuries do sometimes occur.

Who is in Charge?

It's important to find out who is in charge of the study and where it's being conducted. Reputable scientists working at reputable institutions are more likely to perform beneficial, important research safely. Research hospitals, typically facilities affiliated with universities, have oversight groups called institutional review boards. Their job is to make sure that all the work done under their auspices is ethical and scientifically sound, and that adequate procedures are in place to ensure that the patients taking part in experimental treatments understand as well as possible what they are getting into.

What is the Study Testing, and How is It Designed?

Find out exactly what is being studied and the strategy for studying it. Get the person in charge (the lead investigator) to sit down with you and explain it, including just how you fit in. Many studies have a controlled, randomized, double-blinded design. In a drug study, *controlled* means that some of the participants are assigned to an experimental group; that is, they get the active drug being investigated. The others are assigned to a control group, who receive either an inactive placebo (which can't be distinguished from the active drug by appearance or any other readily discernible characteristic) or a current standard treatment disguised to look like the experimental treatment drug, for comparison purposes.

If this assignment to groups is carried out randomly, it is called *randomized*. That doesn't mean that every other patient goes to one group or the other, or some such simple assignment scheme. Randomization is a statistically coded procedure that ensures that there will be a valid random distribution of study participants to the groups.

If the study is *double-blinded*, neither the doctors taking care of the patients nor the patients themselves know who is getting the active drug. As noted above, the assignment is coded, and the code isn't broken until the study is completed or there is some other reason to stop the study.

If there is known to be an effective treatment that prevents harm to the afflicted person, as is the case in rheumatoid arthritis, systemic lupus erythematosus, and many other diseases, it is unethical to deny the most effective known treatment to the control group.

Is There a Safety Committee?

Look into the administrative framework of the study. Is it being conducted at a single institution or at multiple institutions (multi-center)? Is there a safety committee of disinterested parties whose job is to break the code periodically to determine whether a safety issue exists that may require early termination of the study? An example would be a high incidence of some apparent side effect in the experimental group or a definitively better outcome in the experimentals than in the controls, providing an early answer to the experimental question. Especially in multicenter trials, no one center may have enough information to recognize that a trial should be stopped early.

Who is Funding the Study?

Find out who is funding the study and what their interest in the outcome may be. Sources of funding could include the National Institutes of Health, a private foundation, or a pharmaceutical or device-manufacturing company. Will the results be published even if they are negative? Failure to publish negative results tends to bias opinion in favor of effectiveness of the studied intervention. Unfortunately, many scientific journals are not interested in publishing negative results, but the investigator should make a good-faith attempt to publish results whether they are positive or negative.

What's in the Consent Form?

Pay close attention to the consent form. Normal procedure is that someone connected with the study should go through the consent form with you point by point, allowing all the time you need to get all your questions answered. In particular, you should make sure that you understand what happens if you have a side effect that results in additional medical expenses. Who pays them? The consent form should also contain a clear statement that you can remove yourself from the study at any time without jeopardizing your ability to continue to receive standard care for your arthritis. Some studies also have a "crossover" provision, which enables controls to receive the active medication (at no charge for a specified time) at the end of the study period if they so desire. When you understand all this, you can sign—or decline to sign—the form, giving your informed consent.

Appendix 2

Drug Equivalency Table
(Currently Available Drugs)

Generic Name	Brand Name(s)
abatacept [AH-buh-TAH-sept]	Orencia
acetaminophen [uh-SET-uh-MIHN-uh-fuhn]	FeverAll, Tylenol
ACTH [AY-SEE-TEE-AITCH]	H. P. Acthar Gel
adalimumab [aah-duh-LIM-you-mab]	Humira
allopurinol [al-lo-PURE-uhn-all]	Aloprim, Zyloprim
anakinra [aah-nuh-KIN-ruh]	Kineret
auranofin [or-AN-uh-fin] (oral gold)	Ridaura
azathioprine [ay-zuh-THIGH-uh-prin]	Azasan, Imuran
celecoxib [SEL-uh-cox-ib]	Celebrex
choline magnesium trisilicate	Trilisate
chondroitin sulfate [kon-DROYT-'n SUHL-fate]	Chondroitin sulfate
ciprofloxacin [sip-roh-FLOCKS-uh-suhn]	Ciloxan, Cipro
colchicine [KOHL-tschuh-seen]	Colchicine
cyclobenzaprine [sigh-klo-BEN-zuh-preen]	Flexeril
cyclophosphamide [sigh-klo-FAHS-fuh-mide]	Cytoxan, Neosar
diclofenac [dye-KLO-fen-ak]	Arthrotec, Cataflam, Solaraze, Voltaren

diflunisal [dye-FLOON-uh-sall]	Dolobid
doxepin [DOCK-suh-puhn]	Sinequan, Zonalon
d-penicillamine [DEE-pen-uh-SILL-uh-meen]	Cuprimine, Depen
etanercept [ee-TAN-ur-sept]	Enbrel
ethambutol [eh-THAHM-byou-tohl]	Myambutol
etodolac [EE-toh-DOH-lak]	Lodine
febuxostat [feh-BUX-uh-stat]	Adenuric (Europe only)
fenoprofen [FEN-o-pro-fuhn]	Nalfon
flurbiprofen [FLOOR-be-pro-fuhn]	Ansaid, Ocufen
folic acid [FOH-lik ASS-uhd]	Sold under the generic name
glucosamine [glew-KOH-suh-meen]	Glucosamine
hydroxychloroquine [hi-DROCKS-ee-KLOR-uh-kwin]	Plaquenil
hylan G-F 20 [HIGH-luhn] (also known as hyaluronate sodium derivative)	Synvisc
ibuprofen [eye-byou-PRO-fen]	Advil, Motrin, Nuprin, Reprexain, Vicoprofen
indomethacin [in-do-METH-a-sin]	Indocid, Indocin
infliximab [in-FLIKS-uh-mab]	Remicade
isoniazid [eye-soh-NYE-uh-zid] (frequently called INH)	Isoniazid, Nydrazid
ketoprofen [KEE-toh-pro-fuhn]	Oruvail (old name: Orudis)
leflunomide [luh-FLEW-nuh-muhd]	Arava
loperamide [lo-PEAR-uh-mide]	Imodium
meclofenamate [MEK-loh-FEN-uh-mate]	Meclofenamate (old name: Meclomen)
meloxicam [mehl-OCKS-uh-kam]	Mobic
mesalamine [meh-SAHL-uh-meen]	Asacol, Canasa, Pentasa, Rowasa

mesna [MESS-nuh]	Mesnex
methotrexate [meth-oh-TRECKS-eight]	Rheumatrex
metronidazole [MEH-troh-NIDE-uh-zohl]	Flagyl, Noritate
nabumetone [na-BYOU-muh-tone]	Relafen
naproxen [na-PROCK-sen]	Aleve, Anaprox, Naprelan, Naprosyn
omeprazole [oh-MEP-ruh-zohl]	Prilosec, Zegerid
ondansetron [awn-DANCE-uh-trawn]	Zofran
piroxicam [peer-OCKS-ee-kam]	Feldene
prednisone [PRED-nuh-sone]	Deltasone
probenecid [pro-BEN-uh-sid]	Probenecid
pyrazinamide [peer-uh-ZIN-uh-mid]	Pyrazinamide
rifampin [ruh-FAM-puhn]	Rifadin
rituximab [ruh-TUX-uh-mab]	Rituxan
salsalate [SAL-suh-late]	Disalcid, Salflex
sulfasalazine [suhl-fuh-SAL-uh-zeen]	Azulfidine
sulindac [SUHL-uhn-dak]	Clinoril
temazepam [teh-MAZ-uh-pam]	Restoril
tolmetin [TOL-meh-tuhn]	Tolectin
warfarin [WAR-fuh-rin]	Coumadin

Appendix 3

Glossary

Acute phase reactants (APR)
Common, nonspecific blood tests for inflammation. Sedimentation rate and C-reactive protein (CRP) level are the most frequently used. When elevated, the interpretation is that there is inflammation somewhere in the body.

AIDS
Acronym for acquired immunodeficiency syndrome, a disease caused by the human immunodeficiency virus (HIV). This virus destroys certain blood cells that play an important role in immunity (T-helper cells), leading to reduced ability to resist certain types of infection.

Amyloidosis
Disease caused by deposition of protein-containing material in numerous organs (kidneys, liver, heart, among others), impairing their ability to function. Amyloidosis typically occurs in people with long-standing inflammatory diseases such as rheumatoid arthritis or tuberculosis.

Antibodies	Circulating proteins produced by white blood cells called lymphocytes, which are elicited by and bind specifically to foreign proteins or polysaccharides called antigens, leading to destruction or clearance of the latter from the body. Antibodies are one of the body's main specific (immune) defenses against infection. Immunization leads to production of specific antibodies.
Antimalarial drugs	A class of drugs effective against the organisms that cause malaria. An example is hydroxychloroquine.
Antimetabolic drugs	A class of drugs that inhibit cellular replication and reproduction. Often used to treat cancers or to suppress the immune system. An example is methotrexate.
Aplastic anemia	Reduced levels of red blood cells caused by very low blood cell production in the bone marrow. May be accompanied by low white blood cell and platelet counts, a condition known as pancytopenia.
Arthralgia	Pain in joints.
Arthritis	Inflammation in joints.
Aseptic necrosis	Localized bone death, usually near a joint (especially the hip, shoulder, or knee), often caused by high-dose corticosteroid treatment. Also called avascular necrosis.

Autoantibody	An antibody (see antibodies) against components of your own body. Examples include rheumatoid factor, antinuclear antibody, anticardiolipin, and many others.
Autoimmunity	A condition in which the immune system inappropriately attacks your own tissues and organs, thereby causing disease, either through autoantibodies (see autoantibody) or other immune modalities.
Avascular necrosis	Localized bone death, usually near a joint (especially the hip, shoulder, or knee), often caused by high-dose corticosteroid treatment. Also called aseptic necrosis.
Bamboo spine	Fused spine in advanced ankylosing spondylitis, with a typical X-ray appearance that resembles a bamboo branch.
Birefringence	Polarized light transmission property of certain crystals in which the light beam is rotated to make the crystals visible against a black field produced by viewing microscopically through crossed polarizing filters (polarized light microscopy). Aids identification of uric acid crystals (gout) and calcium pyrophosphate dihydrate (CPPD) crystals (pseudogout) in synovial fluid.

Bone marrow	Tissue in the center of many bones, where blood cells are manufactured.
Bone spurs	Overgrowth (hypertrophy) of bone at sites of irritation, typically seen in osteoarthritis.
Bouchard's nodes	Bony protuberances at the proximal interphalangeal (PIP) joints, often seen in osteoarthritis of the hands (see proximal interphalangeal joints). Named for Charles-Joseph Bouchard (1837–1915), a French pathologist who described this phenomenon.
Bursitis	Inflammation in a sac of synovial fluid outside a major joint that normally cushions the rubbing interface between large muscles and bones produced by movement of the joint. Most common at the shoulder (subdeltoid or subacromial bursitis), hip (trochanteric bursitis), and the medial aspect of the knee (anserine bursitis).
Carpal tunnel syndrome	Numbness, often accompanied by pain, in the thumb, index finger, and long finger, due to pressure on the median nerve at the wrist. Frequently occurs in rheumatoid arthritis, but can be seen in many other conditions as well.

Cartilage	Fibrous tissue, commonly called gristle, that acts as a shock absorber in joints. Formed from a protein (collagen), glucosamine, and chondroitin sulfate.
Chemotherapy	Treatment with drugs that kill or arrest the reproduction of cells. Normally used to treat cancer, but also used in autoimmune (see autoimmunity) diseases to suppress the immune system.
Chondroitin sulfate	One of the components of connective tissue, especially bone and cartilage (see glucosamine).
Chronic fatigue syndrome	A condition of unknown cause characterized by extreme fatigue for more than six months, often accompanied by impairment in short-term memory or concentration; sore throat; tender lymph nodes; muscle pain; multijoint pain without swelling or redness; headaches of a new type, pattern, or severity; unrefreshing sleep; and postexertional malaise lasting more than 24 hours.
Complication	An unexpected, adverse effect of a disease or treatment. Amyloidosis and carpal tunnel syndrome are complications of rheumatoid arthritis. Aseptic necrosis is a complication of corticosteroid treatment.

Corticosteroid	A class of drugs structurally resembling and mimicking the effects of hydrocortisone, the principal hormone produced by the adrenal cortex (outer layer of the adrenal gland). The most commonly used corticosteroid is prednisone.
C-reactive protein (CRP)	A protein produced by the liver and released into the bloodstream when there is active, acute inflammation somewhere in the body; for example, in the joints of people with arthritis.
Culture	A laboratory test for infection that consists of growing and identifying a germ (bacterium, fungus, or virus) from a sample of body fluid in an appropriate medium. For example, culturing synovial fluid (see synovial fluid) enables us to diagnose infectious arthritis.
Cyclooxygenase (COX)	An enzyme that enables the formation (synthesis) of inflammatory chemicals called prostaglandins.
Cytokines	Chemicals, produced by cells in response to a stimulus, that act on target cells, resulting in a biological effect. An example is tumor necrosis factor-alpha (TNF-alpha), produced by antigen-stimulated lymphocytes, acting on inflammatory cells, resulting in inflammation.

Disease-modifying antirheumatic drug (DMARD)	A class of drugs that, when used to treat rheumatoid arthritis, suppress the disease effectively enough to slow or prevent joint damage. The most widely used example is methotrexate.
Distal interphalangeal (DIP) joints	The outermost joints of the fingers (see figure C-1).

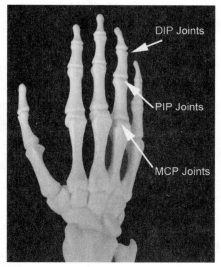

Figure C-1: Skeletal model of a hand, showing the locations of distal and proximal interphalangeal joints and metacarpophalangeal joints.

Erosion	In arthritis, local bone loss at the margin of a joint, as seen on X-ray. Erosions indicate significant damage to cartilage and bone.

Fistula

An abnormal channel from a site of inflammation to the skin surface, through which inflammatory fluid can escape. Fistulas (sometimes called fistulous tracts), from the intestine to the skin surface near the anus are common in Crohn's disease.

Giant cell arteritis (GCA)

Inflammation in the walls of medium-size arteries, most typically the temporal arteries, sometimes accompanying polymyalgia rheumatica (PMR). So named because of the presence of "giant cells" with multiple nuclei in the areas of inflammation. Carries a high risk of visual loss.

Glucosamine

One of the components of connective tissue, especially bone and cartilage (see chondroitin sulfate).

Gluten

A protein found in wheat products, to which people can become allergic.

Heberden's nodes

Bony protuberances at the distal interphalangeal (DIP) joints, often seen in osteoarthritis of the hands (see distal interphalangeal joints). Named for English physician William Heberden (1710–1801), who described this phenomenon.

Histocompatibility (HLA) antigens	Genetically determined proteins on cell surfaces that act as foreign antigens when organs are transplanted from one individual to another unless there is a match between the two individuals.
HLA-B27	A histocompatibility antigen usually found in people with ankylosing spondylitis, reactive arthritis, and some other seronegative spondyloarthropathies.
Immunosuppressive drugs	Pharmaceuticals that suppress immune responsiveness. Often used to treat autoimmune diseases.
Inflammation	The body's reaction to many injurious agents. It is generally characterized by aggregations of cells attacking the injurious agent and in the process causing swelling, redness, warmth, and tenderness. It is the main process involving the joints in arthritis.
Informed consent	A formal agreement, signed by a patient or a patient's legal representative, to undergo a procedure, to share protected medical information, or to participate in research, acknowledging that the potential risks and benefits have been satisfactorily explained. For participation in clinical trials, informed consent forms must be approved by the institutional review board of the sponsoring institution.

Interleukin (IL)	A cytokine (see cytokines) produced by lymphocytes acting on other lymphocytes and inflammatory cells. Designated by number: IL-1, IL-2, and so forth.
Iritis	Inflammation of the iris (colored portion) of the eye. This term is often used interchangeably with uveitis, or inflammation of the uveal layer of the eye, of which the iris is a part.
Koebner's phenomenon	Formation of an inflamed track along the course of a light scratch on the skin. Named for Heinrich Koebner, a 19th-century German dermatologist who described this phenomenon, which is seen in psoriasis and adult-onset Still's disease.
Metabolic syndrome	The combination of central obesity, high blood pressure, insulin resistance, and abnormal blood lipids. Also called metabolic syndrome X.
Metacarpophalangeal (MCP) joints	The knuckle joints at the bases of the fingers (see figure C-1).
mg	Milligram(s).
Monoarticular	Affecting a single joint. An example of monoarticular arthritis (sometimes called monoarthritis) would be an attack of gout in one joint of the big toe or an infection in one knee.

Monoclonal antibody	An antibody (see antibodies) produced by a single clone of plasma cells (the cells that produce antibodies). Such antibodies are generally manufactured in tissue culture and harvested for use in treatment (for example, the anti-TNF inhibitor infliximab) or laboratory testing.
Myalgia	Muscular pain.
Nonsteroidal anti-inflammatory drug (NSAID)	Class of drugs that reduce inflammation by inhibiting an enzyme (cyclooxygenase) responsible for synthesis of inflammatory chemicals called prostaglandins. These drugs are not chemically related to hydrocortisone; thus the term nonsteroidal.
Oligoarticular	Affecting a small but unspecified number of joints. Synonymous with pauciarticular.
Ophthalmologist	Physician specializing in diseases of the eye and their surgical treatment.
Optometrist	Practitioner (doctor of optometry, or O.D.) specializing in nonsurgical treatment of eye problems; generally focused on testing and fitting for glasses or contact lenses.
Pauciarticular	Affecting a small but unspecified number of joints. Synonymous with oligoarticular.

Physiatrist	Physician (M.D. or D.O.) specializing in physical medicine (the use of physical treatments for musculoskeletal and neurological problems) and rehabilitation.
Physical therapist	Practitioner trained to supervise exercise and the use of modalities such as heat, hydrotherapy, and massage, among others, to relieve musculoskeletal problems.
Polyarticular	Affecting a large but unspecified number of joints.
Prostaglandins	Chemicals derived from 20-carbon fatty acids under the influence of cyclooxygenase enzymes, many of which have inflammatory effects.
Proximal interphalangeal (PIP) joints	The innermost joints of the fingers, between the metacarpophalangeal and distal interphalangeal joints (see figure C-1).
Psoriasis	A common skin disease characterized by a scaling, sometimes itching, red eruption, typically distributed on the scalp, elbows, knees, and areas around the umbilicus (belly button), anus, and ear canals. Often accompanied by damage to the fingernails and toenails.
Psychiatrist	A physician specializing in the diagnosis and treatment of mental and emotional disorders, using the full range of therapeutic modalities, including drugs.

Psychologist	A Ph.D. practitioner specializing in the diagnosis and treatment of mental and emotional disorders, using nonmedical therapeutic modalities such as psychotherapy.
Recombinant DNA technology	Laboratory methods of manipulating DNA (the chemical structures that contain genes) at the molecular level. These techniques underlie the scientific field of molecular biology.
Rheumatism	A nonspecific term that generally refers to aching and pains in joints and muscles.
Rheumatoid factor	An autoantibody (see autoantibody) that reacts with a normal blood protein called immunoglobulin G (IgG), forming antigen-antibody (immune) complexes. Immunoglobulins are blood proteins that contain all antibody activity. IgG is one of five classes of immunoglobulins (IgM, IgG, IgA, IgD, and IgE) in humans.

Rheumatoid factor is found in the blood of 80 percent of people with rheumatoid arthritis, but it is also present in many individuals with other conditions, especially chronic infections.

Rheumatologist	A physician specializing in the diagnosis and treatment of rheumatic disorders, including various forms of arthritis and other inflammatory conditions.
Sacroiliac joint	The joint between the sacrum (the lowest five vertebrae) and the ilia (largest bones of the pelvis). Anchors the pelvis to the spine.
Sarcoidosis	Inflammatory disease of unknown cause resembling tuberculosis. Probably autoimmune in nature.
Scleritis	Inflammation of the white layer of the eye (sclera). Can be destructive, especially in rheumatoid arthritis, if not treated.
Scleromalacia	Softening and possible perforation of the white layer of the eye (sclera) caused by untreated scleritis.
Sedimentation rate	Blood test, the most common form of which is called the Westergren sedimentation rate, that measures the rate at which red blood cells settle in a special tube. Generally expressed in millimeters per hour. Used as a test for inflammation, but can be confounded by a variety of other factors—for example, high blood sugar, anemia, and low or high blood proteins.

Sign	Evidence of disease that can be observed (such as a swollen joint). Contrasts with symptoms, which are subjective and can be reported only by the patient (pain in a joint).
Sjögren's syndrome	The combination of dry mouth, dry eyes, and often arthritis. Can occur as a primary condition or a manifestation of some other disease such as rheumatoid arthritis, systemic lupus erythematosus, or scleroderma.
Spondyloepiphyseal dysplasia	Hereditary malformation of the vertebrae and extremities, resulting in short stature with short trunk and short limbs. Can lead to early development of osteoarthritis.
Symptom	Subjective evidence of disease that cannot be observed but can be reported only by the patient (such as pain in a joint). Contrasts with signs of disease which can be observed (such as swollen joint).
Syndrome	A group of symptoms and/or signs that occur together, either as a primary condition or as a secondary feature of various underlying diseases. An example is carpal tunnel syndrome, which can occur secondary to rheumatoid arthritis, myxedema, amyloidosis, multiple myeloma, repetitive trauma, etc.
Synovial fluid	Fluid within a joint.

Synovitis	Inflammation of the joint lining, called the synovium.
Temporal arteritis	Inflammation of the temporal arteries, generally characterized by the presence of so-called giant cells and often used synonymously with giant cell arteritis (GCA). GCA (see giant cell arteritis) may affect the walls of any large or medium-size arteries—most typically the temporal arteries—and sometimes accompanies polymyalgia rheumatica (PMR).
Tender point	Point of muscular tenderness in fibromyalgia at 18 typical locations.
Tendinitis	Inflammation of a tendon. Also spelled tendonitis.
Tophus	Aggregation of monosodium urate (MSU) crystals, usually under the skin, resulting in a lump that can be felt and/or seen, in gout.
Trigger point	Point of muscular tenderness in fibromyalgia at 18 typical locations. Also called tender point, the preferred term.
Tumor necrosis factor-alpha (TNF-alpha)	Cytokine (see cytokines) critical to inflammation in many rheumatic diseases, especially rheumatoid arthritis. So called because TNF-alpha is also responsible for the breakdown of tumor cells induced by an immune response against a tumor.

Uveitis	Inflammation of the uveal (pigmented) layer of the eye.
Valgus deformity	Generally in reference to the knee: knock-kneed deformity in which the axis of the leg is displaced laterally from the axis of the thigh.
Vasculitis	Group of diseases characterized by inflammation of the walls of blood vessels. Classified by the size of vessels involved, whether they are arteries or veins, and the nature of the inflammation.
Xanthine oxidase	Enzyme responsible for the breakdown of purines from the nuclei of dying cells to uric acid. Can be blocked by the drug allopurinol, used to reduce the concentration of uric acid and urates in blood and joints.

Appendix 4

Resources

Books and other sources of the printed word are wonderful, but they have one major drawback: once the last word is written, they begin to go out of date. And few types of information become obsolete faster than medical information. As Thierry Poynard and colleagues wrote in a fascinating article entitled "Truth Survival in Clinical Research: An Evidence-Based Requiem?" published in the *Annals of Internal Medicine* in 2002, the half-life of medical truth is about 45 years. Therefore about half of what we "knew" to be true 45 years ago, we now "know" to be false! That's why it is so critically important to have sources of information that are continuously updated and corrected.

Fortunately, in the modern era we have the Internet, a source of information that is capable of being updated as frequently as necessary to keep it current. Although the Internet is a rich resource for current information, it can be a mixed blessing, since not everything on the Web is equally credible or current. There is no central clearinghouse or quality control mechanism for Internet information that ensures its currency or correctness. For that reason, a bit of guidance for using the Internet should be helpful, and I will attempt to provide it here.

If you enter just the word *arthritis* into the Google search engine, the result is 40 million "hits" in 0.37 second! Narrowing the topic to *rheumatoid arthritis* reduces the yield to 8.05 million references. Phenomenal as that is, and while there may be a great deal of useful information buried in such results, unless a person has a lot of time to sift through such a massive data dump, along with the expertise to critically evaluate it, it's not particularly helpful.

Instead, I suggest going to trustworthy sources of information and seeing what they can tell you about the topic of interest. A few such institutional sources include:

- Cleveland Clinic: *my.clevelandclinic.org.* Then click *A* and scroll to "Arthritis" or any other letter, and scroll to the specific disease; for example, *R* for rheumatoid arthritis.

- Mayo Clinic: *www.mayoclinic.com.* Then click *A* under "Find It Fast" and scroll down to "Arthritis."

- Arthritis Foundation: *www.arthritis.org.* This web site is user-friendly and aimed at non-physicians

- American College of Rheumatology: *www.rheumatology. org.* The ACR Website is aimed mainly at professionals. It is of limited utility for consumers, but disease classification criteria may be of interest.

- Centers for Disease Control and Prevention: *www.cdc. gov.* Then click *A* at the top of the page and scroll down to "Arthritis."

- National Institute of Arthritis and Musculoskeletal and Skin Diseases: *www.niams.nih.gov.* Then click *A* under "Health Information Index" and scroll down to "Arthritis."

- National Library of Medicine/PubMed: *www.pubmedcentral. nih.gov.* If you are looking for the most up-to-date information on a very narrow topic and don't mind wading through some technical language, you can go directly to the scientific literature via the Medline database, maintained online by the National Library of Medicine. Access to this database is free to the public. It catalogs all articles appearing in the peer-reviewed medical literature throughout the United States and most of the rest of the world. Using the PubMed search engine, you can search the database by topic, author, year, journal, or various combinations of these criteria, resulting in a list of references that meets the conditions you set. You may have to go to a library to actually get the articles you find, but the results are often worth it. (A somewhat simpler way is to use the Google Scholar service, at *http://scholar.google.com*, which not only returns the publications you are looking for but also gives the number of times each reference has been quoted in the scientific literature. This is a rough indication of the credibility or importance of the source.)

- Also check out the websites of universities with respected medical schools, such as Harvard and Johns Hopkins. The details of looking through these websites may change without notice.

There are literally thousands of other websites of varying value purporting to contain reliable information about arthritis and related conditions. Beware of those that promote unusual treatments for which the main evidence is found in testimonials. You should check with your physician before trying anything you read about on such websites. As I mentioned at the beginning of this book, the most directly accessible source of medical information at your disposal is your physician. He or she can help you find the information you are seeking, give you an assessment of its credibility, and, just as important, determine its applicability to your situation.

Acknowledgments

I wish to acknowledge that I received considerable help in bringing this book to reality. Gloria Mosesson, our consultant, who assisted us a great deal in the early days of the Cleveland Clinic Press, suggested that I write it and gave me a lot of early encouragement. Peter Studer, head of the Cleveland Clinic's Department of Scientific Publications, read every chapter and made many helpful suggestions. I owe a great deal to Kathryn DeLong, the indomitable editorial director of the Cleveland Clinic Press, who is one of the most optimistic souls I have ever had the pleasure to meet; she and Shannon Berning of Kaplan Publishing are in great part responsible for the survival of much of the Cleveland Clinic Press, including its educational mission, in its reincarnation as a part of the Kaplan Publishing family. In addition, I would like to thank editors Judy Knipe, Allyson Peltier, Kim Bowers, and Patricia Romanowski, without whose insightful recommendations and support this book could not have come into existence in its present form. Finally, I could never have done most anything without the help of my trusty, longtime assistant, Kathleen Maruschak. She is one in a million.

Index

About the Author

John D. Clough, M.D., was born in northwestern Iowa and grew up in Silver Spring, Maryland, a suburb of Washington, D.C. He received B.S. and M.D. degrees from the George Washington University, and in 1965 went to Cleveland Clinic to begin his postgraduate training in internal medicine. In 1967 he returned to suburban Maryland and began a three-year term as a commissioned officer in the U.S. Public Health Service at the National Institutes of Health. There he pursued studies in immunology in the metabolism branch of the National Cancer Institute ur direction of Dr. Warren Strober.

In 1970 he returned to Cleveland Clinic to complete graduate training and joined the rheumatology departm staff member in 1971. He started the Special Immunol oratory for investigation of autoimmune disorders in headed that laboratory until 1990. He was appointed ch the Department of Rheumatic and Immunologic Diseas a post that he also held until 1990. He was appointed director of the Division of Health Affairs at the Clevelan 1990, an administrative post that he held until 2004. position to become publisher of the Cleveland Clinic tion that he held until his retirement at the end of

Dr. Clough is a fellow of the American Colle and the American College of Rheumatology. F the Ohio Public Health Council, and he sits on Ohio Hospital Association, the Academy of land and Northern Ohio, and the Center fo is immediate past chairman of the board School Settlement. He is married and ha grandchildren. He lives in Gates Mills, (